THE MOON IS
A MOTHER, TOO

THE MOON IS A MOTHER, TOO

IS A

TOO

Rituals and Recipes for a Magical Pregnancy,
from Conception to Birth—and Beyond

EMILIA ORTIZ

A TarcherPerigee Book

tarcherperigee

An imprint of Penguin Random House LLC
penguinrandomhouse.com

Most TarcherPerigee books are available at special quantity discounts for bulk purchase
for sales promotions, premiums, fundraising, and educational needs. Special books
or book excerpts also can be created to fit specific needs. For details, write
SpecialMarkets@penguinrandomhouse.com.

Library of Congress Cataloging-in-Publication Data

Names: Ortiz, Emilia (Mental health advocate and healer), author.
Title: The moon is a mother, too: rituals and recipes for a magical
pregnancy, from conception to birth—and beyond / by Emilia Ortiz.
Description: New York: TarcherPerigee [2024]
Identifiers: LCCN 2023052921 (print) | LCCN 2023052922 (ebook) |
ISBN 9780593543429 (trade paperback) | ISBN 9780593543436 (ebook)
Subjects: LCSH: Pregnancy—Religious aspects. | Moon—Religious aspects.
Classification: LCC BL627.59 .O77 2024 (print) | LCC BL627.59 (ebook) |
DDC 133.4/46—dc23/eng/20240416
LC record available at https://lccn.loc.gov/2023052921
LC ebook record available at https://lccn.loc.gov/2023052922

Printed in the United States of America
1st Printing

Book design by Shannon Nicole Plunkett

CONTENTS

This book is dedicated to my children, in both the spirit and physical realms. Without you, I would not be a mother. You initiated me into the path of motherhood and make every day a ceremony of its own. You have my eternal gratitude.

INTRODUCTION

People tend to think of ceremony or ritual as being a singular event and not one that is ongoing. Pregnancy and parenthood challenge that idea by opening the doors for us to live in ritual and ceremony on a daily basis. In many cultures, pregnancy is considered one of the most sacred and spiritual times in a person's life. When a child is born, so is a parent. Carrying and creating life builds a bridge between the spiritual realm and the physical. That bridge is you. Being the link for a soul to make its transition into a physical form is no easy task. As we are on a journey of being pregnant, the soul we're carrying into this realm is on a journey, too, one that doesn't end once the child has been born. It goes far beyond that. Children remain linked to the spiritual realm, and when supported properly can maintain this connection in a way that also supports them. After all, gifted adults were once children, too.

This book is my humble offering to anyone embarking on this journey (or assisting someone through it), from pre-conception to raising these tiny humans/ future ancestors, whether it is your first time or one of many. With knowledge I have gained over the years from personal practice and experience, self-education and research, and teachings from both elders and my spirit guides, I have put together resources to help you at each stage along the way. They include recipes, herbal allies, ritual baths, accounts of my own spiritual experiences with pregnancy, affirmations, wisdom from elders in my life, and more. Think of this book as a guide, and the voyage to and through pregnancy as a national park; there are many trails you can take to arrive at your destination. Some intersect, giving you the option of changing course midway. Use this guide to navigate the path you embark on, but feel free to venture onto another whenever you need.

Remember this as you make your way through these pages: Certain parts may not resonate with you or be for you, and this book is not meant to cover everything under the sun. There's always more to learn. Take what you need, leave what you don't. Always consult your doctor and birth team before working with herbs—and remember, this book is simply another tool in your toolbox of support for your journey. This doesn't replace medical advice or intervention.

A few notes before we dive in. Throughout this book, I mention using prayer or praying. I understand that many folks do not like the concept of prayer because of its association with organized religion. However, prayer has existed in every culture, for ages. It is not owned by a particular institution, religion, or practice. It is something we all have access to—if we choose to tap into it. Prayer is not only a form of connecting with a higher power or petitioning one, it is a way of reaching out to our ancestors, nature, the elements, the cosmos, and more than we may ever come to have words for. It is powerful, and it is one way of putting a life force behind our intentions, hopes, and dreams. It's best to phrase the prayers I suggest yourself. This is because the prayers that have the greatest impact are the ones that are from your heart. So, any time I mention prayer, I encourage you to speak from your heart. Speak life into your intention and the assignment you are giving it. To know the power of prayer is to know the power you have within and the power of the divine that you place your trust in.

Ritual can mean different things to different people, and that's okay. Some rituals are the things we do to unwind from the day and prepare for bed—much like when we help our little ones with taking a bath, putting on cozy pajamas, and reading a story or singing a lullaby to help them make their way to dreamland. Others may involve candles, prayer, and more. All are valid and serve the purposes they were made for.

When it comes to herbs, unfortunately not everyone has access to a well-stocked botanica or apothecary. With this in mind, I have shared herbs that are typically widely available, with only a few exceptions. So while there are, of course, many more herbal allies that you can explore (and that others may suggest), this book focuses on what is accessible, whether you are in a small town or a big city. Most of the ingredients I share can be found in the grocery store or made at home. The internet might seem to have what you need, but unless you have a reputable source, I advise caution when purchasing herbs for healing, medicinal, or supportive use online. You want to be sure what you're purchasing is what is listed and that it is produced with safe processing practices (to avoid mold, pesticides, and other contaminants), and I tend to find brick-and-mortar stores to be more reliable on this front.

There are different reasons we may encounter difficulty with becoming pregnant. There are different reasons why we may encounter difficulty with carrying to term and so on. Often with pregnancy it is believed that your course of action should be tailored to your personal circumstances. As I've often said, something may be medicinal, but that doesn't mean it's *your* medicine. I encourage you not only to personalize what is shared in the book but also to seek out support beyond this book for your journey. You're deserving of it, in all ways.

As with most things in life, take what you need and leave what you don't. While this may seem like one of the biggest mountains you have set out to climb in your lifetime, you are more than capable of making it to the top. Remind yourself in moments of doubt: you've got this.

CHAPTER 1

PRE-CONCEPTION

A common practice throughout the Caribbean is to go out and bathe in the first rain of May. Some will collect it and bottle it up for later use in spiritual baths. It's believed to hold fertile energy, good luck, and cleansing and healing properties. It isn't uncommon to see people collecting the water or bathing in the rain as it pours down. While this isn't a practice exclusive to the Caribbean, the connection is important for the story I'm going to share.

Many years ago, I had a dream about a friend of mine. In this dream, I saw her dancing in the rain, her face filled with joy and excitement. Then I saw her pregnant in her mother's living room, surrounded by flowers and the people she loved most, with a soft green light washing over her. When I woke up, I immediately called to tell her about it, as I believe that pregnancy dreams are never to be dismissed. She laughed and brushed it off, because while she knew what I see in my dreams tends to come to fruition (as with many dreams), especially regarding new life and death, a baby was not on her to-do list. I reminded her, "I'm only the messenger and you can do with this information what you choose, but be mindful."

A little while later, she shared a video on social media of her dancing in the rain. It happened to be the first rain of May in the Dominican Republic, where she was visiting. I wrote her jokingly that I'd be starting my preparations for the baby shower. We both had a good laugh, and she mentioned that her family members had told her about women bathing in the first rain of May in hopes of becoming pregnant. I told her, "Listen, either a baby is on the way or you'll be birthing a new project"—though I knew in my gut which it would be.

A month or so went by, and she called me and said, "I have to start listening to you, because why am I pregnant now?" It wasn't planned, it just came to be. And yes, she had her baby shower in her mother's apartment. As I look back, I still can't help but laugh. That baby was determined to let her know it was coming into this world one way or another. Sometimes pregnancy requires planning and effort, sometimes it doesn't.

NOT EVERY SEED
WE SOW WILL GROW

When trying to conceive, we can get so caught up in the timelines of others. We see friends, family, even people we barely know who seem to get pregnant without trying. It seems to just happen for them, while it can feel like it is taking forever or is impossible for us.

Our timelines always differ from everyone else's, but that doesn't make it hurt any less. The act of releasing expectations, surrendering to the process, is easier said than done—especially while still making an effort to be intentional about conception. How do we find our rhythm? How do we flow with this process? There is no one-size-fits-all solution, and that can be the hardest thing to accept. It is the first step, though, of how our children come to be. In another way, it's a lesson in parenting: things don't always go as planned and we aren't the only person in this. A child is their own person, with their own plans, which is something we have to both respect and work with. Like when they learn to walk, we can provide guidance, support, and someone to catch them should they stumble—but they have to take the steps on their own.

We often hear parents say, "You were just a twinkle in my eye," when telling their children about how they came to be. Before they are conceived in the physical plane, children are realized in our minds and in the spiritual realm. Even the thought of wanting to conceive can sometimes plant that seed in the universe. For some, this takes a long time to become anything; for others, it grows into the opportunity to adopt, or it may eventually grow into a wanted pregnancy (this includes surrogate pregnancies as well).

We plant the seed, but ultimately many factors come into play. We're not the only party involved, and all paths to parenthood are unique—which makes sense, because our life paths are one of a kind, and so are those of our children. None of this makes for a 1 + 1 = 2 situation. This is frustrating (it would be so helpful if there were a fail-proof formula!), but the first step is understanding that your experience won't look like anyone else's, so there's no point in comparing—especially since we don't know what others have gone through to get here. These differences shape us into the type of parent we'll be. Your journey here didn't look like everyone else's, so why would your time raising children look like everyone else's?

The way forward is not linear, and this can be hard to embrace. Sometimes our most careful plans miss the whole picture or don't account for other factors. This is where spirit can come in and transform our expectations. The spirit of the child may have certain things they agreed to before coming here. Shifts in how they come into this world may need to occur. Surrendering to that is part of the process, but it is far from easy to do.

While my child's father and I were trying to conceive, it seemed like everyone around me was getting pregnant like it was nothing. It was so hard for me to experience joy for my friends while sitting with the grief I experienced each time I got my period. There were baby showers I attended with a heavy heart and a fake smile on my face. There were baby showers I didn't attend at all. I didn't want to take away from anyone's joy at such a special time. Some people are able to think to themselves, *It's happening to those around me; soon it'll be me.* I couldn't get myself into that perspective, although I did try. What helped me most was being real with myself, setting boundaries, connecting with nature, and practicing self-kindness during the waves of feelings—and we'll get into how to do all of that. Being real about how I felt was important because fronting like I had faith when it felt like the most difficult task wasn't going to do anything for me. It wasn't going to change my circumstances or make me feel better while I waited. I'd only be masking my true emotions. Eventually all masks have to come off, so it's better to never put one on.

WORKING WITH
MOON CYCLES

Throughout this emotional roller coaster, the moon was one of my greatest allies for retreating, releasing, building myself back up, and riding the changes in the tides of my emotions. In the times I felt most full, it illuminated what I was praying for, and it was my guiding source in the times I felt deep uncertainty. If you find yourself having difficulty at any stage of the conception process, consider looking to the moon for support. You can even just talk to her.

Working with the moon is powerful, especially in regard to conception. The moon possesses a special feminine energy, one that can manipulate the tides and influence our menstrual cycles. The end of our cycle each month is the shedding of the lining that was built to keep a baby inside and safe, which your body releases if there is no baby. The moon helps pull that down. It's only right that it would help in the process of a seed being planted, holding tight instead of shedding the lining.

After all, the moon is a mother, too.

The new moon is a time for setting intentions and new beginnings. Here is a simple ritual you can do to work with this phase of the moon.

New Moon, New Intentions

Florida water*

A white beeswax taper
  candle

Handful of dried
  patchouli leaf

Handful of dried rose

Handful of dried raspberry leaf

A heat-safe dish

A pen and paper

*Florida water is a spiritual cologne that can be found in botanicas, metaphysical stores, Latine groceries, and bodegas. Some practitioners make their own Florida water that can be purchased through them as well.

1. First, cleanse your space using your preferred method, whether that's an energetic room spray, or smoke from burning dried herbs or resin incense on a charcoal tablet. Move about the room, getting in the corners especially, and pass the smoke over yourself and the area you'll be working in. If using a spray, spray throughout the room, over yourself and your work area (see page 97 for my favorite sprays). Open the windows so there is a way for the energy you're cleansing from yourself and the space to make its exit. Call upon your honorable guides and ancestors. Thank them for their presence and protection. Ask that they shield you and assist you in this working. Cleanse the candle with some Florida water to remove any energies that it came in contact with previously. Next, sprinkle each of the herbs on the heat-safe dish. Mix them together. Gently roll the candle in the

herbs. Form the leftover herbs into a circle on the dish, leaving room in the middle for the candle.

2. Write down on the paper the intentions that you are setting. For example, you could set the intention of calling in fertile energies, calling in the ability to embody the essence of fertility, or simply becoming pregnant. Honor what is in your heart and feels best. As you hold the candle, channel your energy into it. Charge it with your energy and intentions. Speak them as you see the energy flowing from you into the candle. When you feel this is complete, set the paper under the heat-safe dish and melt some of the wax underneath the candle to help it stick to the dish. Next, light the candle while speaking your intentions. You can follow this up with prayer, or if you don't feel comfortable with prayer, focus on visualization. Visualize yourself as already being pregnant, giving birth, playing with your future child. Visualize it all as if it has come to be. Do this until the candle burns down. Thank your ancestors and guides for their assistance. Dispose of the remnants of your candle work. Keep the paper in a safe place until your intentions come to be. You can either keep this in a memories box or bury it in your yard-space (keeping it close to home).

....

Working with Saint Anne for Fertility Support

Saint Anne is Mother Mary's mother and is the patron saint of a few things, including motherhood, pregnancy, and fertility. She is relatively simple to work with and only requires a few things.

White altar cloth

Florida water

1 Saint Anne seven-day candle

Saint Anne oil

1 glass of fresh water

Sweets of your choosing (candy or pastries)

White flowers of your choosing

Cleanse your space and prepare it with the altar cloth. Then cleanse the seven-day candle by running it under cool water and then rinsing it with the Florida water. Trim the wick just a bit. Place a few drops of the oil onto the top of the candle (on the wax). Place the candle and glass of fresh water on the surface, along with the white flowers and sweets. Light the candle and then center yourself. Recite the prayer on the candle. If there is no prayer on the candle, either say a prayer from the heart or purchase a prayer card so you can easily continue to pray to Saint Anne on a daily basis. Include your petition of asking to become pregnant, to grow your family, and to be blessed with the opportunity to have a child. Let the candle burn all the way down. Do not blow it out. If you must, snuff it out and relight the following day at the same time. Recite the prayer when you relight it. Pray each day that the candle is lit until the candle has burned down. Additionally, you can repeat this ritual throughout your pregnancy to ask her for protection and a safe, smooth delivery.

....

CALLING IN AND COMMUNICATING WITH THE BABY'S SPIRIT

Calling in and communicating with the baby's spirit is an important part of connecting with your baby before their arrival. Take time out of each day to center yourself and speak directly to your baby's spirit. If you already have a name in mind, you can use that, or you can use a phrase, such as "baby of mine," if that is better suited. Tell them all the things you want to share with them. That could be how excited you are or what you're looking forward to doing with them. I shared with my baby how much I already loved them, how excited I was at the thought of being their mommy. I shared my hopes and dreams for them, which consisted of their experiencing joy, love of all kinds, and the ability to make their dreams a reality. I spoke of my commitment to protecting, loving, nurturing, and enjoying life with them. Calling in the baby's spirit is like illuminating a lighthouse in the night. It can guide them to you. While some ships find their way even in pitch-darkness, it doesn't hurt to shine a beacon their way.

HERBAL SUGGESTIONS
FOR YOUR JOURNEY

Herbs are what I consider to be members of our earthly family. Like family members, herbs can be wonderfully supportive allies throughout our lives. It is important to note that while there are many different forms of herbalism, one common philosophy is that herbalism is not a one-size-fits-all practice. The herbal suggestions shared throughout this book are suggestions for a reason. They are a nudge in the direction of connection, or reconnection, with our herbal family members. Consider consulting an herbalist or a homeopathic doctor for protocols using these herbal suggestions.

HERBAL SUGGESTIONS

- **Red raspberry leaf infusion:** Tones the uterus and prepares the womb space for pregnancy and labor. Fill a small tea ball with dried red raspberry leaf and place in a mug. Boil 8 ounces of water and pour over. Allow to steep for 3 minutes. Sweeten with honey to your liking.

- **Maca:** Helpful in balancing hormones and energy levels. This is to be consumed by capsule or powder. Consult an herbalist for your specific dose.

- **Rose tea infusion:** A heart tonic for when you need extra self-love and care. Fill a small tea ball with dried rose and place in a mug. Boil 8 ounces of water and pour over. Allow to steep for 3 minutes. Sweeten with honey to your liking.

- **Rue:** Rue can be a powerful ally in cleansing your womb to support a future pregnancy, but preparations and doses vary from person to person, so consult an herbalist before introducing it into the mix. This is not to be consumed if you may be pregnant, to avoid miscarriage.

- **Lemon balm infusion:** An ally for those with anxiety about the process who need some assistance with calming their nerves. Fill a small tea ball with dried lemon balm and place in a mug. Boil 8 ounces of water and pour over. Allow to steep for 3 minutes. Sweeten with honey to your liking.

- **Castor oil pack:** Supports your uterus in preparation for conception. Castor oil packs can be used on various parts of your body to support your fertility when you hope to become pregnant. Soak a piece of cotton cloth (or a wrap made specifically for this process) that can easily cover your pelvic area in castor oil or pour about 1 tablespoon of castor oil directly onto the cloth. Then apply to your pelvic area. Leave on overnight or for at least an hour. Doing this daily can be exceptionally helpful, but weekly is also supportive if that better fits your schedule and lifestyle. Stop if you suspect you may be pregnant.

AFFIRMATIONS

Affirmations are a simple way to continue your workings and support your mental health. While they do not replace therapy or make everything sunshine and rainbows, they can be effective in helping you along the path. You can write them on Post-its and place them throughout your home, then repeat them whenever you spot one during the day. You can recite them in the mirror to begin and/or end your day: doing it in the morning brings that energy into the day, and in the evening, it closes out your day in a positive way. However you choose to integrate affirmations into your life, I suggest reciting them three times in a row each time.

Using affirmations has been shown to have a beneficial impact on your brain, and for most people, it takes around twenty-eight to thirty days to adopt a new way of thinking—so keep it up. (It may take longer or even less time, because we're all different.) Work with the affirmations shared at the end of each chapter in a way that is most doable for you as far as consistency goes. Consistency is key!

Speaking them into your life can not only change the energy around you, it can help change your perspective and mind. It works if you work it.

AFFIRMATIONS

- My pregnancy journey is unlike any other; that is what makes it sacred.

- I am deserving of support on my terms.

- What others may want or need does not define my needs.

- The timeline of others does not reflect my timeline. That is okay.

- Each chapter in my story is simply that, a chapter; it is not the end of the story.

CHAPTER 2

CONCEPTION

E very act of conception, in both the mind and the physical realm, is a ritual in which what was once created becomes a creator.

We have energetic exchanges every day, from a handshake to an intense conversation. These energetic exchanges create things, from a sense of comfort to new discoveries. There is something magical in the act of fertilization, whether it happens in the privacy of your candlelit bedroom, in a doctor's office, or across the country with a surrogate. Do not be discouraged if your experience is different; it does not make it any less divine or special. We take on the role of creator any time we put something into the world, whether it's another life or a work of art—and, really, who's to say they're not the same?

For years before I had a baby, my plants were my children. One of my oldest is an aloe. My mom gifted her to me when she was a small seedling. In her journey to me, she was crushed in the car when she fell off the seat. When they arrived, my mom said that if the plant died, she'd get me another, but to see what I could do. I cleaned her up and tended to her day by day—talking to her, sending energy to her. She not only made a full recovery, but shortly after, she had three babies.

Plants have a lot to teach us; they'll talk if you listen. My aloe's message was that I would one day have babies of my own, but much like hers, the journey would not be perfect. There would be bumps along the way. There would be scrapes and bruises. I had spoken life into her and tended to her wounds, and I would have to do the same for myself. She made it clear that the journey to and through motherhood would break me open in ways I could never have imagined, in ways no one could fully prepare me for—not even her. This wasn't a warning but a truth that every parent learns in their own time, no matter how "naturally" parenthood comes to them.

Conception was the first challenge to my expectations. I thought it would be *One, two, three, I'm pregnant!* Over the years, I had received countless readings with my elders that included a warning that if I wasn't trying to get pregnant, I needed to mind my P's and Q's when it came to protection. My ob-gyn said there was no reason to believe I was anything less than "fertile Myrtle." None of it made sense. More important, I was hurting.

In time, I learned that the roadblock was bigger than whether I was a ready vessel. You've probably heard the saying "We can plan, but God decides." Whether you believe in a higher power or not, we all know that things don't always work out as anticipated. Nevertheless, it hurts, especially when it seems there is no reason they shouldn't come to pass. Sometimes life works out in ways far better than we could have ever planned. Other times, it is so painful and heavy we find ourselves in a state of despair.

I did eventually conceive, and each time, it was a whirlwind of emotions and sensations. My concept of time shattered, and at moments, I felt like the baby was already there, even though I couldn't hold them in my arms. I could feel the two souls coexisting in my body. There was a sense of grief for the life I had known, but there was also joy beyond comprehension. There are no words in the human language to encapsulate that kind of alchemy.

I also experienced miscarriage, so each pregnancy brought grief and anxiety, and difficulty staying present. I tried to remind myself that in this world multiple things can be true at once. I could be overjoyed, and cautious about getting ahead of myself. I could celebrate and honor this magic while also honoring my pain from before. I could hold space for the trauma that resided in my body and praise this new life that was in my body. You don't have to abandon the bad or compromise the good. They can both be present.

RITUALS AND PRACTICES

Ritual can be a part of our lives in a way that supports us as we navigate our days. Ritual is personal, and whether it's your morning cup of coffee or listening to that special song on your way home from work to help you close out your day, there is power in it. This is extra crucial to remember when you're on your journey to conceive. Continue your personal daily rituals and incorporate some new ones that are specific to this experience. I've suggested a few below to prepare you for the different stages of pregnancy and beyond.

Visualization: This is beneficial for reasons beyond manifesting. It will allow you to prepare for everything from connecting with your baby while they're in the womb to feeling empowered during labor to ironing out the details for your postpartum recovery. Whatever your goals, it is good to get into the practice now. No matter how you plan on conceiving or having a baby (IVF, IUI, surrogacy, adoption), visualization can be a powerfully supportive tool.

To begin, focus your mind's eye on your desires—whether it's seeing yourself as pregnant, giving birth, or holding a baby—as though they have already come to fruition, like you did in chapter 1 with the new moon. If you want to take this a step further, visualize your goal, as if it has already happened, during orgasm. The energy your body is generating and releasing into the universe in that moment can be channeled to call in what you desire.

If you plan to conceive via IUI or IVF, I encourage you to use visualization during the process, as well as rituals, such as candle work, anointing yourself with a fertility oil, and doing spiritual baths before your appointments. If you are working with a surrogate, consider seeing if she is open to any of the practices shared in this book, and do them together. You can visualize connecting with the baby and sending loving energy to the baby, even from a distance. The baby knows you are their parent, even if you aren't carrying them in your physical body.

Altar: An altar is typically a space that is consecrated and dedicated to a specific energy. This energy can take on the form of deities, ancestors, spirit guides or a spiritual court, and specific intentions. An altar can be simple or elaborate, but when creating one, always use discernment and follow the protocol associated with the altar's purpose.

Candles: Candles do more than add ambiance and set the mood. They give light to our intentions and prayers. Consider lighting a candle when you are setting intentions or saying a prayer, as outlined in chapter 1. You can also get a seven-day candle specific to your desire to place on your altar. Add a few drops of patchouli oil or another fertility oil by using a dropper to add directly to the wax on the top (avoiding the wick). Sprinkle herbs, such as dried patchouli or dried rose, on top instead of rolling the candle in the herbs like you would a taper candle, then keep it lit for the entire seven days, saying a prayer or stating your intentions each day at the same time. If you must put it out, snuff it out—do not blow it out—then relight it at the same time the next day. (Unlike with your birthday candles, it is considered bad practice to blow out candles being used for intentional workings.)

Helping something grow: When I became pregnant with my firstborn, I was growing a lot of cucumbers and calabazas (kabocha squash, some also use this term for pumpkin). I talked to them daily; I poured love into them like water. My harvest was bountiful in more ways than one. These particular veggies are associated with fertility and can invite fertility into the home if you nurture them. For anyone wishing to conceive, try planting them. As they grow, they'll draw in fertile energy. Then eat the fruits of your labor.

When I shared this tip on social media, many wrote me with similar experiences. Some became pregnant during the growing season, some after the harvest. It's a simple act that can make all the difference.

If you're limited in space but have a balcony, you can still grow cucumbers in a container. Make a trellis for them to grow up, and help the vine to climb when it is long enough; the plant will do the rest. Unless pollinators come up to your balcony, encourage that fertile energy by taking the pollen from the male flowers with a clean makeup brush and dusting it inside the female flowers. (The female ones have a little bud under them.) Just like us, nature can use some helping along. You could try this with a pumpkin or kabocha squash, but it may be difficult considering they need to sprawl out a lot more.

Another way to bring abundant energies into your home is by keeping a rose of Jericho (associated with abundance, fertility, and protection, especially for birthing parents and their babies) in a bowl of water. Change the water regularly. You can sprinkle yourself

daily with water from the bowl to enhance your fertility as well. Some midwives used to bring them when
going to deliver a baby, to bring on an easier labor (as
the plant rehydrates and opens, so does the cervix);
some midwives used them to predict when the baby
would come by divining with the plant.

Calling it in with herbal allies: Many herbs are associated with or used in fertility work. If you're not comfortable consuming them, you can work with plant
allies topically and on an aromatic level. A few of my
favorites for aromatic and topical use are red clover,
patchouli, geranium (white geranium), and bee balm/
wild bergamot.

Light a patchouli or bee balm/wild bergamot candle
or burn patchouli incense before being intimate to fill
the room with fertile energies, or anoint yourself with
patchouli oil before your IVF appointments. Try having your partner give you a massage with geranium
oil, and focus on visualizations of conceiving or talk
about how excited you both are to become parents.
Use a red clover spray and call on the plant's ability
to help with fertility. There are many ways to connect
with plant allies for support. Do what you're most comfortable with.

Another way to work with herbal allies is to place
a bundle of horsetail in your pillowcase or elsewhere

in the bedroom, such as under the mattress. Having daffodils in the bedroom can also support conception. If you're choosing to dress a seven-day candle, place a few echinacea seeds, patchouli, and geranium on the top, then anoint it with a few drops of a fertility oil, such as patchouli, bee balm, rose, rose of Jericho, or a blend from a botanica before burning. If you're using a taper candle, dress it with the herbs, then scatter the echinacea seeds on the plate around it.

If you are comfortable consuming herbs and wish to explore teas or infusions, consult an herbalist for proper dosage and inquire about working with red clover, nettles, oat tops, red raspberry, or rue (for pre-pregnancy use only to help cleanse the womb).

Unfortunately, there are instances where we did not consent, and the act of creation is traumatic. Some don't wish to move forward, some do. Some have the option to not move forward, and some don't. Whatever someone chooses is to be respected. There is no right or wrong way for the survivor to move forward; there is simply what they feel is best. If this is resonating for you, my advice is to seek support, no matter what decision you make. You deserve to be supported through your process and experience, wherever your journey takes you.

HERBAL SUGGESTIONS

- Patchouli: Use patchouli cologne in baths or wear it to call in fertile energies. It can also be sprayed in your bedroom or added to the washing machine when you wash your sheets for the same purpose.

- Red clover: Make an infusion by filling a mesh tea ball with red clover, then steeping it in 1 to 2 cups of boiling water for 20 minutes. Add honey to taste.

AFFIRMATIONS

- I have faith that my personal process of becoming a parent will be preparation for supporting my future child's journey.

- I am surrounded by fertile energy that will bring me the opportunity to become the parent I dream of.

- I am deserving of grace in this process; I will extend the grace and compassion I give to others to myself in this time.

CHAPTER 3

FIRST TRIMESTER

L ike all of pregnancy, the first trimester is different for everyone. Some have no symptoms, while others have every complaint under the sun. Like most, I was nauseous and beyond exhausted. I also had such intense hip and pelvic pain that I needed to seek outside help.

Recharging so I could refill my own cup was one thing. I had embraced falling asleep before seven p.m. and taking multiple naps a day (intentionally or not). Allowing someone else to tend to my physical body, opening up to the idea of someone I didn't know touching me, was something I hadn't often done.

During a meditation one day, I had a vision of my body being out of whack and misshapen from the baby that was growing. Then I saw a figure of light shaped like a woman putting my body back the way it needed to be. I heard the word "chiropractor" and looked up whether that was even an option during pregnancy. I found a woman in Brooklyn who specialized in chiropractic work for pregnant people. It was one of the best things I did for myself during those nine months. Just as I had seen in my vision, I had a rotated pelvis, among other alterations, that my body was making to compensate for the growth of the baby. The human body may be intelligent by design, but that doesn't mean the execution of its tasks is without flaw. The therapeutic work allowed the energy to flow properly again and assisted my nervous system in communicating with the rest of my body. The relief was instant and felt so damn good. I saw her throughout my pregnancy. For the first time in my life, I was committed to someone who only poured into my physical body (aside from my nail tech, that is). I was expected to relax, release, be filled up, and leave feeling better than when I arrived.

If you are struggling with something, whether it's the aches of your physical body or an anxious mind, seek out help. You deserve to find a healer who can move with you through these exciting and uncertain months, whether that's a chiropractor, massage therapist, acupuncturist, psychiatrist, or therapist. If you're like me, you're used to handling everything yourself—

but it's not just about you anymore. Set yourself up to be the best, most loving parent you can be by extending that love to yourself first.

SETTING BOUNDARIES

Too many mothers begin neglecting their own needs early on, but it doesn't have to be that way. The first trimester is a time for setting boundaries because it sets the tone for the rest of the pregnancy and into parenthood. Be choosy with what you give your time to, who you take advice from, who you allow to touch you, what you're okay with doing. Practice making yourself clear, and you'll be prepped for when your baby arrives—and, as they grow, for showing them by example how to establish healthy boundaries.

Consider wearing colors that are reflective, which can prevent you from absorbing energies that weigh you down. Saying no can also be an act of protection. A baby bump is not an invitation to be touched, no matter how many people may act like it is. If you don't want people touching your belly, say that and be firm; it doesn't matter if it's your mother-in-law or your best friend. If anything doesn't feel comfortable, honor that. Consent goes beyond sex. If they still don't get it, ask them how it would feel if you went around rubbing their stomach. Sometimes we need to prompt empathy by asking people to put themselves in our shoes. Remind them—and yourself—that boundaries aren't about punishing but are set with the intention of preserving the relationship you have.

Here's a simple exercise to practice setting protective boundaries. Visualize yourself surrounded by an ultraviolet bubble. This bubble is a protective force field keeping any negative energy from penetrating. Feel its strength and ability to let any energy directed toward you bounce right off. As you do this, say this affirmation out loud three times: "The people I come into contact with today are not entitled to my energy." Sit with the image as long as you like, then close out the exercise by saying, "So it is spoken, so it shall be." Practice setting firm boundaries with whoever you come into contact with that day, even over small things, keeping your energy balanced and neutral and not giving it where it shouldn't be given. While for many exercises you want to get into a certain setting, this is one you can do at any moment to reinforce your energetic boundaries.

I also advise my friends and clients to try a popular psychology-based approach, which is the gray rock method: When you have to engage with difficult people, be like a gray rock. Do not give anything that can lead the conversation to something personal. Avoid topics that can become heated; try to focus on topics like the weather, or something else more neutral. If they bait you, don't take the bait. Center yourself and remember to be as boring and neutral as a gray rock. Be as boring in your response as possible, e.g., "It's interesting that you feel that way," or even just, "Oh, okay." Don't give them anything to feed off. While at first they may try even harder to provoke you into a response, just continue to be a gray rock. You'll walk away feeling just fine instead of drained.

SUPPORTING NAUSEA AND OTHER SYMPTOMS

Being pregnant is a special time in life, but it doesn't mean that you're comfortable. Nausea is the classic telltale sign, of course, with frequent offerings to the porcelain god and finding yourself repulsed by the smell of things you once loved. That favorite perfume or those cooking onions now bring only misery. You don't have to accept being completely miserable in your pregnant body, though. Seek out professional help, especially if your symptoms are severe, such as in the case of hyperemesis gravidarum, which is persistent nausea and vomiting that can lead to hospitalization, dehydration, weight loss, lightheadedness, and feeling faint.

On the positive side, nausea is often considered a sign of a healthy pregnancy—basically, it's like a hormone hangover. (Although, if you aren't experiencing nausea, there's nothing to be worried about, so congratulations! Enjoy! Pregnancy can be taxing enough; it's always a win if you're not feeling the physical ails) While you may be inclined to only nibble on crackers, there are other ways to find relief, including the following:

- **Bodywork, such** as massage, acupuncture, and chiropractic adjustments.

- **Eating grounding foods,** such as root vegetables, which have the double action of preventing constipation (which contributes to nausea and is often a symptom of the first trimester) and grounding you energetically. Carrots, potatoes, and yuca have a deep connection to the earth and can root you and soothe your stomach. See pages 39–42 for my favorite root veggie recipes.

- **Eating small meals** after your nausea subsides.

- **Increasing your protein intake:** Whether it is plant or animal based, you need more protein to grow that baby. The body is intuitive that way; what the baby needs, you do, too.

- **Ginger and/or citrus:** Everyone claims ginger is the saving grace for nausea, although it did nothing for me. Citrus, specifically lemon, is what did the trick. Lemons and limes balance the acids in our stomach, providing relief. Try hot water with lemon or lime, lemonade/limeade, or even sorbet (the cold can be extra soothing). A trick one of my midwives shared with me is also to scrape off a little from those frozen lemonades they sell in stores if you need something easy. See page 43 for an extra-hydrating citrus pop recipe.

- **Warm baths:** I enjoyed taking baths with lemon slices and ginger. Thinly slice the ginger and slice the lemons like you would for lemonade. Boil 1 gallon of water, pour over ginger, steep for 20 minutes, strain, and add to the tub water (or—let's be real—have your partner or a friend or family member do this). The bath gave me an energy boost and alleviated my symptoms, especially with a cup of Epsom salt thrown in. If you are under the weather, this particular bath blend can get you back on your feet. Note that some say ginger baths are not safe for pregnancy. It is best to consult your doctor or herbalist before taking one.

I admit that I personally subscribe to many superstitions, but there are many around pregnancy that I don't believe in. Many folks will tell you that nausea indicates that you're having a girl, because girls give trouble from the start—or, on the flip side, that boys are easier even when you're pregnant, or some other sexist bullshit. Don't get caught up in it. Your symptoms are not a sign of what's to come with your child's assigned sex, demeanor, personality, health, etc. Do your best not to project onto them before they're even here; give them a chance to show you who they are when they're earth-side.

FIRST-TRIMESTER RECIPES

Yuca with Onions

Yuca is one of my favorite root vegetables. I'm happy to have it boiled with butter, like you might cook potatoes. Olive oil with a little salt sprinkled on top is great, too. Below I've shared two recipes that make use of yuca and are simple but delicious.

1 or 2 (depending on size) peeled fresh yuca, or 6 to 12 ounces frozen yuca, cut into chunks

½ cup avocado oil

1 red onion, sliced thinly

2 tablespoons white vinegar

1 head of garlic, peeled and finely chopped or mashed in a pilon/mortar and pestle

Salt and pepper, to taste

Bring a large pot of water to a boil. Add chunks of yuca. Reduce the heat to medium-low, cover, and cook for 20 minutes or so, until the yuca is fork tender (similar to a potato). While the yuca is cooking, in a separate pan, heat avocado oil over medium heat and add the red onion. Allow it to cook down until translucent, then add the vinegar and garlic. Let the vinegar and garlic get a touch of heat to release more flavor. Remove the yuca from the pot and set aside. Pour the onion and garlic mixture over the yuca. Add salt and pepper to taste.

Note: While many use olive oil for cooking, avocado oil is better for this recipe because of its heat tolerance. If you prefer the taste of olive oil, use ¼ cup of avocado oil to cook the onions and add the olive oil to the mixture at the end, right before pouring.

....

Bacalao con Verdura/Viandas

While many people are most familiar with yuca fries, I grew up with the boiled version. A favorite of my dad's and mine is called bacalao con verdura/viandas, or salted codfish with vegetables— boiled green banana, plantain, potato, yuca, yautia, or ñame (often all of the above, but if you can't get them all, make do with what you can). These two recipes are simple but delicious. (You can also just boil chunks of yuca, as you would with potato, and add some butter if you need something that's one-two-three.)

1 pound salted bacalao
or pollock

3 green plantains or bananas
(or both)

2 yuca, peeled and cut into
chunks (be sure to remove
the woody center;
sometimes it's easier to do
this after it's been boiled)

1 or 2 yautia, peeled and
cut into chunks

1 or 2 ñame, peeled and
cut into chunks

4 or 5 medium white
or red potatoes, peeled
and cut into chunks

Drizzle of olive oil, to taste

Optional: 1 egg and 1 avocado

Note about ingredients: Some of these can be hard to find if you're not in an area with a Caribbean greengrocer. It's okay to leave out what you can't find, but I'd suggest a base of yuca, green plantain/banana, and potatoes at the least. This is one of those recipes that is really about preference and accessibility. Make do with what you can find, and include as many or as few of the ingredients as you'd like.

Prepare the bacalao by rinsing it to get most of the salt off, then soak it in cold water for a few hours, changing the water once an hour. I typically do about three changes. Fill a bowl or your clean sink with cold water.

Slice the green plantain skin just enough that water can get in and loosen the skin, which makes for easier peeling. Place them in the water and allow to soak for 20 to 30 minutes. Check them with a knife by trying to peel back the skin. (This step is optional but makes it easier.) If using green bananas, wear gloves when peeling them to avoid staining your hands. Once both the fish and the green plantains have soaked enough, bring two large pots of water to a boil. Remove the skin from the green plantains. Add root vegetables to one pot and bacalao to the other. Let them boil until the vegetables are tender and the fish is flaky. The cooking time for this can vary, but start checking at the 25-minute mark. Drain both, and make sure the fish is deboned by checking through with a fork. While they may be sold as deboned, there are often one or two left behind. If you are using the egg, boil it in the same pot as the root vegetables or in a small separate pot if that is easier. Boil until cooked fully, about 8 to 10 minutes, then peel, slice, and add to the plate. If using avocado, cut the avocado in half, remove the pit, and make several slices. Scoop out and add to the plate. Serve the rest by putting the fish and vegetables in a bowl and pouring olive oil over everything. Add salt if necessary, but taste first; often it isn't needed because the fish is already salted. This is different from the stewed version of bacalao and gentler if you're experiencing morning sickness, because it isn't acidic.

....

Maple-Glazed Carrots

These are a quick and simple way to get the grounding energies of root vegetables into your next meal, and they're a delicious side dish to serve with something savory to balance out the sweetness, such as baked chicken.

5 or 6 medium to large
   carrots, peeled and sliced
   into medium coins

½ tablespoon maple syrup

2 tablespoons butter
   (or nondairy substitute)

Fill a medium pot with water about a quarter of the way. Bring it to a boil and add the carrots. Cook for 15 minutes or until tender; strain. Return them to the pot and add the maple syrup and butter. Cook on medium heat, stirring occasionally, until the consistency becomes syrupy. Another option, if you're feeling more indulgent, is to cook the carrots in half a stick of butter first—no water—until it's all absorbed. Then add the maple syrup and cook until thickened.

....

Watermelon and Lemon Ice Pops

1 small watermelon, rind removed, cut into chunks

½ small lemon

1 set of ice pop molds (silicone works best)

Optional: 1 tablespoon honey or agave

Run the watermelon chunks through a juicer, or puree in a blender and then press through a mesh strainer. Squeeze or use a citrus juicer to juice the lemon. In a large bowl, combine the lemon juice with the fresh watermelon juice. If you're adding in honey or agave, do so now. Pour into the silicone molds and place a stick in each. Freeze. Grab one whenever you feel the nausea coming on.

....

Mocktails

While these recipes will nourish you (and make you feel like an adult with a drink in hand) at any stage in pregnancy, they can be particularly helpful in the first months, when liquids may go down easier. They also have energetic benefits, because they all integrate protective plant allies for extra goodness.

Creamy Lemon Elderflower Soda

Lemon, coconut, and elderflower have cleansing and protective correspondences on an energetic level. On a physical level, lemon helps soothe nausea. Blueberries are protective as well—and bring all the flavors together.

1 cup white sugar

1 cup freeze-dried blueberries

½ small lemon

1 to 2 tablespoons condensed coconut milk (or condensed dairy milk), to taste

8 ounces sparkling elderflower lemonade

Ice

Add sugar and blueberries to a coffee grinder or food processor. Blend until well combined. Now you have blueberry sugar. Juice the lemon. Dip the rim of a cup in the lemon juice, then dip it in the blueberry sugar to line it. In a separate cup, add condensed coconut milk and about 2 tablespoons of sparkling elderflower lemonade. Stir with a spoon until the milk has dissolved. Taste—it should be just slightly overly sweet because it will become toned down when you add the ice and lemonade. Pour into the garnished cup. Add ice, then fill the rest of the glass with sparkling elderflower lemonade. Stir gently and enjoy.

....

Virgin Mule

Lime is cleansing, mint offers some protection and cleansing, and ginger amplifies both effects. These ingredients also provide nausea relief, giving you multiple benefits as well as refreshment.

1 cup sugar	Ice
1 lime	4 ounces ginger beer (nonalcoholic)
A few fresh mint leaves	

Prepare the simple syrup: Combine the sugar and 1 cup of water in a pot and cook on medium heat until the sugar is fully dissolved. Allow to cool before use.

Juice lime and place juice into a cup. Add 1 tablespoon of simple syrup. Take a few mint leaves and clap them between your hands a couple of times before adding to the cup. Add in ice and ginger beer. Stir gently and enjoy.

....

Rosemary Peach Breeze

Rosemary is protective energetically and is safely consumed as a food. The peach is refreshing and uplifting, while the lemon offers cleansing properties.

Handful of fresh rosemary sprigs (about 6 to 10), plus one for garnish

1 cup sugar

1 small lemon

3 fresh peaches, 1 chopped and 2 juiced (or 1 fresh peach, chopped, and 4 ounces store-bought peach juice, not concentrated)

Splash of soda water

Ice

Prepare the simple syrup: Add the rosemary, the sugar, and 1 cup of water to a small saucepan and simmer for 15 to 20 minutes, or until the sugar is fully dissolved and the liquid has changed to a pale golden yellow from the release of tannins in the rosemary. (Note: some pans may cause the liquid to look darker than it is.) Strain, set aside, and allow the liquid to cool completely. Chop up a peach. Juice the lemon, then add 1 tablespoon lemon juice (or more to taste), 1.5 tablespoons of the rosemary simple syrup, a splash of peach juice, and the soda water to a cup. Add in the chopped peaches and ice. Give a gentle stir. Garnish with a rosemary sprig.

....

Lady Lavender Mocktail

Lavender helps with sleep, is protective, and brings in peaceful energy. The lemon and lime offer cleansing, protection, and a sense of calm, and it will settle your tummy. If you want to make this one to wind down at the end of the day, consider adding a tablespoon of magnesium powder.

½ tablespoon store-bought lavender syrup

1 tablespoon lime juice

Ice

6 ounces carbonated lemon water

1 lavender sprig, for garnish

Add the lavender syrup and lime juice to a cup. Stir until fully combined. Add the ice and the carbonated lemon water. Stir gently and garnish with the sprig of fresh lavender.

....

As someone with a Taurus moon, I am all about the good eats and how food can connect to our emotions and provide a sense of comfort. For me, what we eat and what we drink can be medicine of many kinds, including for the heart. There is an aspect of ritual behind the process of cooking or making a mocktail. Pour your love, good thoughts, and intentions into it. Keep this in mind as you consider how ritual can play a role in your first trimester (especially since this time may leave you feeling exhausted).

FIRST-TRIMESTER RITUALS

A Visualization for Connecting with Baby

Nourishment is not only about what food we eat but about what energy we put into ourselves. One of the ways I connected with my baby from the start was this exercise, which you can try for five minutes a day to begin with. Lay your hands on your stomach. Visualize a bright green light flowing from your heart, through your hands, to your baby. Feel the love radiating from your heart, surrounding your baby and filling them up. Gradually increase the amount of time that you spend with this each day.

(Re)establish a Relationship with Nature

Nature is a healer, if we are present and open to witnessing her ability to be. Her children share their healing abilities with us, if we are present for them: The wind that carries away stagnant energy and lifts us up with a refreshing breeze. The water, in its many forms, that cools, soothes, and washes away. The plants that lend their wisdom and energy to ease physical and spiritual ailments. The sounds of thunder, songbirds, ocean waves, and rain that vibrate through us and take our pain with them. The earth that we stand on, that centers us, that nourishes our bodies and souls. The light from the sun and moon and stars that wraps us up like a blanket and at the same time acts as a guide through the journey of life. Nature is a healer, but we have to be present and open to receive her gifts. Otherwise, we're just passing through and not honoring all she has to offer.

The beginning of both my pregnancies was in summertime, so I spent a lot of my days in nature, especially at the beach. Getting in the ocean, letting the salt water cleanse and remove any unwanted energy, has always been healing for me. I might be a fire sign, but I am absolutely a water baby. The crashing of the waves, taking anything negative out to sea; stepping out of the water feeling refreshed; and charging up under the rays of the sun have always been my medicine. While I was pregnant, this experience was amplified, and every time I left the beach, I felt better than when I arrived.

If you are pregnant in the warmer months, I highly suggest you get into a moving body of water (ocean or river), if possible. It does wonders for cleansing and balancing energies, not to mention mitigating physical discomfort. Oceans and rivers not only are mothers to many creatures that reside in and depend on their waters for food and shelter, they're mothers to those of us who inhabit this earth, offering lessons of feminine energy and fluidity, power, strength, and beauty. Holding us in times of strife and difficulty, providing us with nourishment for the body and soul. Lending comfort to us, and sweetness. Showing us how destruction, while sad at times, can be necessary and even restorative. Being a model of shape-shifting and resilience. Water, in its many forms, has so much to teach us, if only we are open to learning.

If you're not comfortable in water or don't know how to swim, you can try the simple act of bringing an offering, such as fresh fruit, to leave at the shore as thanks. Speak your thanks out loud. Then sit on the beach, bank, or shore and meditate. Let the water's energy wash over you just by being in what we can consider to be its auric field—radiating out beyond the water's reach. Take in the sea spray or simply the sweetness that a river pours into everything surrounding it. Bask in it, and take it all in.

Connecting with nature during pregnancy lowers your stress levels. It also gives your baby a strong connection to the world they'll come into before they are earth-side—and helps you to stay grounded during the roller-coaster months to come. There are so many transitions that occur in pregnancy, so having a grounding force to visit is essential. When you embody the energy of nature's children, the air will be the wind beneath the wings of your spirit when needed, the earth will center you, the water will cleanse and soothe you, the animals will guide you by example. Be open to taking it in and witnessing the many offerings and medicines that you're shown. It's no coincidence what you are a witness to. Nature's children know what they're bringing to you.

Honor Your Ancestors

Ancestral veneration can be a wonderful tool to support your growing family and you. Pregnancy can feel lonely at times, so remember that you aren't alone. Even if the room appears to be empty, those who came before you are with you. Celebrate with them. Share your concerns with them. Thank them for walking with you. Pray for the elevation of your bloodlines.

Ancestral veneration looks different for everyone. It isn't the act of worshipping your ancestors, it is the act of honoring and loving on them. Lighting candles; playing their favorite songs; leaving their favorite sweets, fresh fruit, or meal in a special place; saying a prayer for the elevation of their spirit; calling on them for support out of respect for their wisdom and strengths. You can do this in whatever ways fit your comfort level. You don't have to include anyone you had a harmful relationship with; you can set boundaries even when someone is gone from the earthly plane. Personalities and energies that people embodied in this lifetime don't magically change when they've transitioned. Which is why this, too, is a form of protection.

Energetic Protection

During pregnancy, not only is your intuition heightened, but so is your energetic sensitivity, which can lead you to be more vulnerable to psychic attack, the evil eye/mal de ojo, etc., the same way your immune system is compromised, making you more susceptible to listeria or even a cold. Options for protecting yourself include the following:

- Working with crystals, such as black tourmaline or jet, by keeping them on your person, at your front door, and/or in your personal spaces. Hold them while you meditate and visualize them creating a protective shield of energy, one that transmutes anything negative sent your way.

- Wearing protective jewelry/talismans (ain't gotta get ready if you stay ready) such as an azabache, hamsa, seven-knot red string bracelet, or peony/peonia-seed bracelet. Avoid the latter if you have small children in the home, as the poisonous seeds fall off as they protect you. You can also try a St. Michael/San Miguel pendant or red waist beads/a red string tied around your waist. These (aside from the waist beads/red string on the waist) can also be used for your baby when they arrive.

- Getting your jewelry blessed steps its protection up a notch and can be essential for its working as protection at all. Priests and priestesses, healers, and energetic practitioners can all bless your jewelry. Sometimes it is a family tradition to have a certain family member bless jewelry, such as a grandmother who is known to pray over the family. There is no one right way of doing this, and each will likely have their own approach. Some will incorporate working with the elements, deities, saints, etc., while others will focus solely on prayer. Work with someone whom you feel is trustworthy, and don't just go with whoever's offerings are the flashiest. Sometimes simpler is better for your personal needs—and sometimes it's not. Listen to your gut.

The first trimester is taxing physically, emotionally, mentally, spiritually. It is part of the beginning of your initiation. It will change you forever. Lean into the different forms of support that exist for you to call on.

Calling on Saint Anthony

Saint Anthony is the patron saint of a few things, but my favorite way to work with him is for finding lost things. Pregnancy brain can have us misplacing things in the wildest of places. Saint Anthony is very helpful with finding lost items; he has also been known to some as the patron saint of those with child. When you are needing some help with finding a lost item, say the following out loud: "Saint Anthony, Saint Anthony, please come around, something is lost and can't be found. Oh, Saint Anthony, I have lost my _____. Please help me find it quickly/return it to me, Saint Anthony." When you find the item, or it's been returned, say thank you out loud to Saint Anthony. There are variations of the phrase that's said. But this is what I have used time and time again, and he always comes through.

HERBAL SUGGESTIONS

- Create a bundle of fresh basil, sage (cooking/garden sage), and rosemary. Use a sweeping motion from head to toe to remove any negative energy. Pray or speak words of affirmation or of being cleansed. When the bundle wilts, you'll know it did the job. Throw it in a garbage can outside of your home. Thank the plants for their assistance before disposing of them.

AFFIRMATIONS

- I trust my body to guide me through this journey and tell me what is needed.

- Creating life is nothing short of a miracle, and so I am a creator of miracles.

- Rest is an act that I am worthy of.

- Birthing on my terms is an act of resistance in the face of medical oppression.

CHAPTER 4

SECOND TRIMESTER

To bear life is an initiation, one of many that life has to offer.

I woke up one Sunday and felt flutters in my stomach. A wave of warmth washed over me as I lay there in amazement. There is no way to describe how it feels to experience those first movements. It isn't butterflies; it's more magical than that. As time went on, those movements helped me to better know my baby, in ways that made their transition so much smoother. It was the foundation of our bond, our connection, that aided me in being able to understand my baby's needs in real time.

Each stage of pregnancy includes opportunities for initiation into motherhood/parenthood. Each one is personal, and sacred to us in our own way. They prepare you not only to birth this tiny human but to birth a mother/parent as well. Embrace your process.

For some, this includes healing wounds around advocacy and finding their inner voice. For others, it means healing their inner child and learning how to be present in the moment.

Once I tapped into my baby's rhythms and nuances, that early understanding of their internal clock was invaluable. I learned quickly, for example, that my baby was generally active in the womb from seven a.m. until about eight p.m. When I woke up in the middle of the night to pee, they would adjust and quickly settle back to sleep. I was delighted to find that the same was true now that my baby was earth-side. Even when they would wake to nurse in the night, they would go right back to sleep after, then wake at seven a.m., same as in the womb. Later, I was prepared for the structure of nap time during the day and knew that each time they adjusted their position at night, it wasn't a call for me to soothe them back to sleep. (It's also why we have stuck to a schedule of winding down starting at seven thirty p.m. and getting to bed by eight or so. The few times we didn't, baby made it clear that the party was over and bed needed to happen now.) Don't worry—if yours is a night owl in the womb, it doesn't mean you're doomed to late nights forever. But having that knowledge will prepare you to better understand how to structure their days and nights.

If my baby was being too active and I couldn't get comfortable, I rocked. I swayed while holding my belly, and soon my little one settled down and I was able to get a nap in. I made sure the way I rocked and swayed felt natural to my body. I was preparing my baby to embrace this movement and associate it with the comfort of the womb.

In order to support our children when they make their transition from womb to earth, we have to remember that they spent nine months in a controlled environment: warm as a Jacuzzi, provided with continuous nourishment, soothed by our heartbeat, protected from the elements. When they emerge into this world of dry air and fluctuating temperatures—where they no longer hear our heartbeat (except when on our chest) and there are strangers, bright lights, and weird smells, and they have to cry and call out for breast/chest or bottle service—there is a shift in the way they are protected; it's an adjustment.

As we discussed in the previous chapter, being in communion with nature and earth energies not only supports your baby but will anchor you through all the hormonal and physical changes you're both going to go through—in pregnancy and beyond. Nature will be an ally, not just for you but for the baby, too.

SECOND-TRIMESTER RITUALS

Grounding into and Honoring Mother Earth

During those nine months, the earth called to me, especially in the second and third trimesters. Her message was to be diligent about grounding as a way of supporting me but also supporting my baby in building a connection to the earth, which would be a guiding force for them as they got older. They'd be called to play and explore, and they'd find peace, wisdom, healing, and shelter from the storms of life in her arms.

Start by going outside and touching your bare feet to the earth, whether that's dirt, grass, sand, or pebbles. That alone can be enough. Expanding on this practice, close your eyes and visualize roots extending from the soles of your feet into the earth. Feel the energetic exchange anchoring you and providing balance. As you feel this, so does your baby.

In the colder winter months, when I wanted to keep my shoes on, I connected with trees instead: hugging them, talking to them, exchanging energy with them, leaving offerings for them.

These actions are simple but powerful. Our ancestors were often barefoot and in nature day in and day out. We have to tend to the disconnect that has occurred. Getting out in nature as much as possible is helpful in reviving this connection, and while big swaths of nature aren't easily accessible everywhere, a tree, patch of dirt, or corner of grass will do just fine. Seek out your local community garden.

If all else fails, get to know a houseplant. Hold the potted plant as you do your daily meditation for protection, grounding, calmness, etc. I suggest an aloe or snake plant that you can place in the nursery or in your bedroom (if your baby will be sleeping there) for protection after they are born. I like clay pots because not only are they better for the plant but they provide grounding energy for you as well.

Another way to connect to the earth for both grounding and cleansing is with mud or dirt. Mud baths are popular at spas for a reason, and you can get all those benefits simply by getting dirty, so to speak. Cover yourself with mud or dirt and visualize any negative energy being absorbed back into the mud as its grounding energy envelops you. Rinse off with cool water. (Avoid getting it in your coochie to prevent infections. For some it may not cause any issues, but we all have different bodies and want to avoid disturbing the delicate individual balance we each have.)

Even in our dreams, nature calls to us. We just have to be open to receiving what is coming through. In the second trimester, my midwives noted that my baby was taking their time turning into the head-down position. While delivering a breech baby without surgical intervention isn't impossible, it is not ideal. I did all the things they recommended to encourage the baby to turn, such as a side-lying hip release. Ultimately, though, nature's spirit has a way of helping things along in unexpected ways.

Midway through my second trimester, I dreamed of dolphins. I was swimming with them, being guided in crystal waters. The sunlight was shining down through the water, illuminating everything below. I could feel the warmth and water washing over me. As I floated, the pod approached my stomach, crowding around and pressing their noses to my belly, whistling and clicking, communicating with my baby. As they did this, my baby moved into the head-down position, performing a somersault inside of me. The dolphins jumped out of the water playfully, in celebration of what had just happened. I smiled from ear to ear and thanked them for their assistance. They continued to play, and I watched in awe until I woke up in the morning. I was feeling at ease and knew it would only be a matter of time before my dream came to be. Nature's spirit had been clear and direct, so I just needed to have faith. Later that day, I was standing in front of my mirror brushing my hair when I saw, and felt, my baby turn into position. It was one of the most wild things

I've ever witnessed—a somersault happening inside of me, just like in my dream. While I knew it was going to happen, it didn't take away from the magic.

Nature's spirit works with us in so many ways and at so many different times in our lives. So many of us are consumed with technology and the day-to-day that it can be easy to disconnect from what really matters. It's okay if it has been a long time since you last were intentional about connecting with nature. She is forgiving if you make the effort. Reaching out during pregnancy allows us to be supported by her, as we were intended to be.

Healing Through Sound

For many years now, I've been a believer in the power of sound, and I made sure to play all the greats for my baby. Some believe Mozart will make their baby a genius. I went with Whitney, Celine, and Mariah, to name a few. The music I chose spoke to my heart and soul, and I wanted to share that. I wanted my baby to hear these artists who could move the soul with their words, their voices. When my baby was three or four months old, they started to sing themselves to sleep, which showed the connection they had built with music. While self-soothing is a taught action and it takes many times being soothed by someone else to learn it, my baby was doing it in their own way, with something that they'd learned to love in the womb—sound.

Embrace the magic of music on your terms. Play songs that you have an emotional connection to, that are culturally significant for you, or that are simply by artists whose voices move you. Pay attention to the lyrics and messages behind them, because as many say, words are spells. This doesn't mean you can't enjoy the genres you love that aren't necessarily kid friendly. You are not limited to soft music or classical music. Just be mindful of incorporating songs with softer topics for balance.

Sound is a powerful tool. Healing sound baths have become more common, and your religious/spiritual practices and ceremonies may include bells, drums, or flutes. These instruments can be used for energetically cleansing people and spaces. Certain instruments can call in spirits at an altar or shrine, or act as a guide for calling a person's spirit back into their body if they have experienced soul loss, when your body and soul become disconnected from each other due to trauma. Deaf people can feel the vibrations of sound, and those same vibrations cause objects to move and dance. This physical representation reveals just a fraction of sound's capabilities, not to mention the mental and emotional impact it brings.

If you want to turn off your streaming and go tech free, try humming instead. The vibrations we generate as we hum stimulate the vagus nerve, which is part of the parasympathetic nervous system, transmitting information to and from the brain and throughout the body. It can positively affect mood, digestion, heart rate, and sensory functions, so doing this for a few minutes several times a day can have a profound impact. When your body is better able to communicate with itself, it completes tasks more efficiently—which is good for baby, too. When the time comes, you can teach your kid this skill to support their process of learning to regulate their emotions.

Now that we're in the toddler stage, my partner and I often play DJ to our little one and, of course, honor the requests that come in—many of which are songs we played while I was pregnant or when our baby was little. My partner is a musician, and we each have experienced the healing abilities of music in our own way. Music and sound have been a saving grace many times in my life. My grief, heartache, and deep depressions have all had a soundtrack (so have my times of joy and bliss), one that helped me to go through the motions and ultimately heal. The words and the artist's talent alone can sometimes be enough, moving energy around and through me, helping me to feel seen by the lyrics.

Modern baby culture focuses on creating baby geniuses, and while intelligence and technical ability are important, so is having a connection to our innate tools for healing, especially in a world with so much pain. We all experience difficult emotions. Being able to lean on your favorite music and restorative sounds can go a long way in getting you through them.

HERBAL SUGGESTIONS

- **Sandalwood incense:** Burning sandalwood will cleanse and bring peace to you and your space.

- **Irish sea moss:** This can be taken in the form of a gel or capsule to provide essential vitamins and minerals to support you, your immune system, and baby.

AFFIRMATIONS

- I wholeheartedly embrace Mother Nature's divine support in my pregnancy.

- I am connected to the earth, and so is my baby.

- I am divinely guided by spirit in all ways, as is my baby.

CHAPTER 5

THIRD TRIMESTER

The third trimester is such an intense time. You feel like a giant pear with reflux and heartburn and a bladder the size of a pea; everything is squished inside; lightning crotch is a thing; you're exhausted but also need to prepare—the list goes on. You may start contemplating how early you can safely serve an eviction notice in hopes of reclaiming your body as your own. I experienced mixed feelings of "I want this baby out now" and "I don't want to risk anything by moving too fast."

At the time, some of my social media followers said that they had been waiting for my baby to come for what felt like forever. While they meant well and were simply excited for me, it brought on a mix of emotions. I was grateful, yes, but I also wanted to yell that I was the one experiencing the pregnancy, going through the symptoms, but more important, waiting. No one wanted to meet that special little someone more than I did. I had spent my whole life waiting for them. There were others who said they wished I would have a Pisces, meaning that my baby would come early. This gave me anxiety, because aside from knowing I wanted an Aries (a Sagittarius mom with an Aries kid is a match made in astrological heaven), I didn't want there to be any issues from an early arrival.

I became adept at quickly blocking people without reading their comments too closely. Whether or not you're on social media like I am, people will make similar comments or ask when you're due every two seconds. Being gentle with and extending grace to ourselves, which can mean firmly setting boundaries with others, is a crucial act of self-care during this vulnerable period. Then you'll have more time and emotional space to focus on what really matters— preparing for labor and postpartum. There are many ways of doing this, but don't be afraid to block or mute anyone on social media (or even in your text messages). As far as what to do in real life, I'd suggest simply reminding them, "I'm doing my best to enjoy this last bit of being pregnant and preparing for labor/the postpartum period. I know you're excited, but I'd appreciate your support in helping me be present for the now." You can also tell them to mind their business if you'd prefer something short and sweet instead.

Establishing a connection with baby while they're in the womb isn't about when they arrive but how. Getting to know them ahead of time can help move them through labor and make the process less traumatic for them (and us). We can do the prep work, write up what seems to be a foolproof plan, hire the perfect birthing team, scout the ideal location, but it can all go out the window for many reasons, including our baby not being on board with some element of the agenda. It's up to us to do our best to create a safe plan and environment but also to allow the baby to lead, or at least have a say in what's going down. This is easier for us to make happen if we have some sort of relationship already. As you prepare your birth plan, check in with your baby. Ask for a sign of what they'd like to happen, speak with them daily, tell them how nice it is outside the womb, share your excitement. Share your plan. Babies and children have a way of not only humbling us but teaching us. If we open up to that reality early on, it's easier for us to work with, rather than against. The third trimester is a testament to that.

If you find that your baby is not in the ideal position, movements such as side-lying hip releases are often recommended. Something that isn't discussed as often is communicating with your baby. While certain movements or positions encourage them to switch theirs, it's mainly out of discomfort, the same way being nudged on a crowded subway by someone who wants you to move makes you move (or go off on them if you're a native New Yorker). In addition to whatever movements you are prescribed by your doctor or midwife, a gentler, more collaborative way to ease baby along is by chatting and checking in with them. It might feel silly or unnatural at first, but keep at it— soon enough you'll hear them talking back, even if it's in a way that only you and they understand. Your special language and ability to understand them when no one else can begins in the womb.

A physical way to connect is by engaging in play with your baby in the womb. Poke at your stomach and make note of where they poke back. More often than not, they're pretty accurate in finding where you just touched them. It becomes a game between you two the more frequently you do it. I always found myself amazed and laughing when I would poke at my stomach and see the movements that followed. These little things prepare you for how to come up with ways of connecting with your child on their level when they're older.

TIPS FOR PHYSICAL
AND ENERGETIC RELIEF

Physical discomfort is almost a given, but there are
some things you can do to try to mitigate it. Some of
these may bring you relief, and some may not. Unfortunately, nothing is one size fits all in pregnancy—not
even maternity clothes.

- **Back pain and body aches:** Try a vapor rub (doesn't
  have to be a specific brand), or as I and many
  others jokingly call it, "la cura." It can be used for
  many things, including congestion relief, nausea
  relief (as aromatherapy), and menstrual cramp
  relief. The menthol is soothing and relieves pain
  in your back. It can even help if you are having
  difficulty sleeping—rub some under your nose for
  aromatherapy, or hold the jar under your nose
  until you fall asleep. Do not rub on your stomach
  or pelvic area. Many vapor rubs contain camphor;
  check with your doctor about the safety of
  camphor use in pregnancy or find a camphor-free
  option if needed.

- **Leg cramps and growing pains:** Try an Epsom salt
  bath, followed by rubbing magnesium oil or spray
  on your calves and legs. Bonus: have someone
  massage it into your legs and feet. You can also

combine this with your favorite lavender lotion for a really calming experience that makes sleeping much easier during this stage.

- **Acid reflux/heartburn:** Try coconut milk or a coconut smoothie (blend coconut milk and coconut meat together) or goat milk. Drink a cup when symptoms occur or as a preventative measure before bed or following your last meal of the day. If you're allergic to coconut, opt for goat milk. If you are allergic to coconut and follow a plant-based diet, go with your preferred milk.

- **Itchy skin relief:** Try pure cocoa butter or shea butter. Slather it on and let it work its magic. Aloe gel and honey are other options, as are lotions or butters infused with chamomile or calendula. If using honey, wash off with lukewarm water and then cold water, without soap.

- **Energy cleanse:** Get a bar of honey goat milk soap from a small business, such as a farm stand, farmers market, soap maker, or goat farm. Wash from head to toe, because moving downward takes away whatever energies you don't need. Visualize a light that encompasses all the colors of the rainbow coming out of the showerhead, washing over you as the water runs down your body, sending all negative energy down the drain. Air-dry. You can also use plain coconut soap as well, with no added fragrance.

THIRD-TRIMESTER PRACTICES
Energetic Nesting

When preparing your baby's room for their arrival, even if you plan on having them in your room to start, think beyond a décor theme. You want to make sure the energy is right, and the third trimester is the time for getting everything ready. From what you wash their clothes in, to how you clean their nursery, to the objects you place in the room, it can all make a difference in your baby's transition. Here are some of my favorite ways to set up yourself and your space for what's to come.

PREPARING THE ROOM

- Aloe and snake plants bring protective energies into your baby's room.

- If you have been feeling a particular animal calling to you during pregnancy, place an image or stuffed version of it in the room. I saw deer throughout my pregnancy, including in places you would never expect to, so I made sure to have one in my baby's room and one in my room to watch over and protect us.

- It is common practice in many cultures to place a prayer card for either your family's saint or a saint of your choosing on the underside of your baby's bassinet or crib to guard them.

- Hang bundles or sachets of dried herbs, such as lavender for protection and peace.

- Place a small glass bowl with water and a camphor tablet in it for spiritual protection (out of children's reach, because if consumed it can be toxic). This should be changed weekly.

Washing Baby Clothes

For newborn clothes, add organic rose hydrosol to the wash. Hydrosols are gentle enough to be used on babies, won't stain clothes, and carry the spirit of the plant. Rose is not only for love, which you want to surround baby with, but for protection, so with each wash, you'll be infusing your baby's clothes with loving care. (Traditionally, homemade rosewater is used, but it can stain clothes.) Spiritual colognes, such as

Florida water, lavender cologne, and agua de violetas, have similar energetic properties, but they can be irritating to a newborn's skin. Use these when your baby is a little older (as opposed to fresh out of the womb) and less likely to have a skin reaction.

Sweet Snacks

Eating dates in the third trimester can encourage a smoother labor, so snack on them regularly (with some protein like a handful of nuts to prevent a sugar spike). If you don't like the taste or texture, try adding them into a smoothie with a protein powder instead. Keep dates on hand after the baby arrives, because they can ease digestive issues and provide the nutrients you need to replenish postpartum as well.

Cleansing the Space

Before my estimated due date with my firstborn, I made sure to clear out the energy of our home so it would be free of anything heavy and filled with sweet, loving vibes. While this is something I do regularly, I switched it up a bit, since I'd be bringing a baby into the home who would be sensitive to smoke and strong scents. I burned onion and garlic skins with the windows open to clear, followed by rose petals for sweeter energies (keeping the baby bedding and clothing packed up outside or wrapped in plastic while doing this). I followed up by dipping a bundle of fresh basil in a mix of holy water and Florida water and sprinkling it throughout the home, from the back to the front, praying as I went. Some people prefer to mop from the back to the front of the house with an herbal floor wash, tossing the water out the front door when finished. This is something I do as well, but I'll admit that at this stage the idea of any extra mopping was exhausting and something I tasked others with. If you feel called to cleanse your space, do what works best for you.

Setting the Scene

If you are having a home birth or plan to labor for a while at home before heading to the hospital or birthing center, set up where you plan to labor and/or deliver, knowing that you may end up somewhere else. Create the ambiance you'll need, which means low or soft lighting (consider leaving all the lights off and curtains closed and using candlelight) and removing any strong smells from the area, which can contribute to nausea during transition. Think about what is grounding for you, what helps you to find your center when you are at your worst, and add those into the mix.

Making a Plan

Your birth team is going to play a key role in your experience, either positive or negative. Consider who brings a sense of calm and peace, who affirms you and who does not. You may want your mother-in-law present; you may not. Either way, stand firm in this decision and don't bend for the sake of others' feelings or desires. They're not going through this—you are. If this feels like something that will be too overwhelming for you, consider asking a friend or your partner to handle any of these conversations, whether via text or phone call. Your doula (if you have one) should embody an energy that you feel confident in, and your midwife or ob-gyn should make you feel affirmed in your ability to do this safely. Any friends or family members who are present should be people you feel will be able to focus on you and not make the moment about themselves. This includes being mindful of whether their own traumas (that you are aware of) may interfere with their capacity to do this. Everyone will have their own role to play, whether that's pain management, tending to the energy of the space, helping you with advocacy, making meals for the team, providing emotional and spiritual support, capturing the magic on camera, or helping you look your "best" in photos and videos (if that is something you're concerned with—ain't nothing to be ashamed of!).

Wherever you plan to deliver, make sure your birth plan includes a list of things you are not comfortable with, and share any trauma with your birth team. Sexual trauma can show up in scary ways during labor, so it's key for your team to be informed and mindful. If you have experienced medical gaslighting or harm, discuss this with them as well. Be as transparent as you can be; this way there will be few to no surprises that arise as far as being triggered goes. It can help you work together and influence how they care and advocate for you.

Thinking Ahead

Padsicles are a game changer in postpartum healing, and making them ahead of time (or delegating a loved one to do it) takes the stress out of it in the moments after birth. Get a few packs of overnight 100 percent cotton maxi pads, a few bottles of witch hazel, and a large bottle of aloe vera gel. Unwrap the pads and place them into a few ziplock bags, making sure not to crowd them. Dump in witch hazel and aloe gel so that the pads are saturated. (I eyeballed this, and it'll work just fine if you do, too.) Pop these in your freezer and use them in your jumbo mesh panties or adult diapers after delivery to help you heal. (I used the latter.) Take it to the next level with herbal supports: steep a tea ball filled with chamomile and calendula, let cool, strain, and pour the liquid over the pads before freezing. This combo can reduce inflammation and provide a calming effect.

RECIPES

These are the kinds of nutrient-dense recipes that you should prep and store before giving birth or task a loved one with making for you. Your body doesn't want cold salad and potato chips right now; to prepare for the hard work ahead, make sure you're getting in plenty of protein, fats, and warming meals.

Stewed Chicken

Typically for this recipe you'd use legs and thighs. These days, I use boneless chicken breast chopped into chunks because it's easy to serve to a toddler. Either is fine!

- 4 boneless, skinless chicken breasts, or 6 legs and 6 thighs, skin on
- White vinegar (to clean chicken)
- 1 head garlic, peeled and crushed or pureed
- 1 yellow onion, chopped
- 1 bunch celery, chopped
- About 5 ounces frozen corn or several fresh chunks of corn on the cob (approximately 10, but feel free to use more)
- 6 medium to large carrots, peeled and sliced
- 6 yellow potatoes, peeled and cut into chunks
- 3 tablespoons adobo
- 2 tablespoons sazón
- 2 tablespoons avocado oil
- 3 tablespoons sofrito/recaito

1 (8-ounce) can tomato sauce

32 ounces chicken broth or chicken bone broth

Optional: Add a few spoonfuls of sugar, to taste, if you prefer a sweeter stew. Traditionally you would add olives, but my household isn't a fan, so I leave them out. You can also add in other vegetables, such as calabaza/kabocha squash or any others you feel called to.

Clean the chicken by rinsing with water, then chop into chunks if using breasts before placing in a bowl (if using thighs and legs, place directly into the bowl after rinsing with water) and pour a ½ cup to 1 cup of white vinegar over it. It should cover most of the chicken—you may need more or less, depending on the bowl you're using. Let sit for 10 minutes. Season the celery, corn, carrots, and potatoes with half of the adobo and half of the sazón. Drain the vinegar from the bowl and season the chicken with the remaining adobo and sazón. Add the avocado oil to a large pot on medium heat. Place the chicken in the pan (skin-side down if using thighs and legs). Turn when browned, and remove when finished browning. If using chicken breast, dump in the chunks and stir occasionally to brown all sides; remove when browned. Add in garlic, onion, and sofrito/recaito. Sauté for about 5 minutes, stirring occasionally. Add the cooked chicken and vegetables. Pour in the tomato sauce. Pour in the chicken broth or bone broth. Add water if needed to fully cover. Cook on medium heat until it begins to bubble. Cover and reduce heat to medium-low. Stir occasionally to avoid sticking. Taste as it cooks (after about

30 minutes), and feel free to add more seasoning or sugar as mentioned. Cook for 1½ to 2 hours. I like mine thick, but if you prefer a thinner broth, cook for less time but until all meat is tender. Serve with white rice and sliced avocado, if desired.

Note: This recipe can be made ahead of time and frozen. Just make the rice fresh.

....

Black Garlic Chicken Soup

This soup is nutrient dense and delicious (with a bonus of some kitchen witchin' courtesy of the protection that garlic brings).

5 boneless, skinless chicken breasts (chopped into medium chunks)

White vinegar (to clean chicken)

6 yellow potatoes, peeled and chopped

6 carrots, peeled and sliced

1 bunch of celery, chopped

5 ounces frozen corn, or 8 to 10 chunks of fresh corn on the cob

2 tablespoons adobo

3 tablespoons black garlic, crushed in a mortar and pestle

2 tablespoons avocado oil

2 tablespoons of sofrito/recaito

6 cloves garlic, crushed

32 ounces chicken broth or chicken bone broth

1 cube chicken bouillon

Optional: yuca chunks (they will continue to soak up the broth after cooking if added), plantain balls, or other vegetables you feel called to toss in

Rinse the chicken breasts with water, then chop into chunks. Put in a bowl and cover with white vinegar (½ to 1 cup, depending on the bowl you use). Let it sit for 5 minutes. Season the potatoes, carrots, and celery with 1 tablespoon of the adobo. Drain the chicken, then season with the remaining 1 tablespoon of adobo and crushed black garlic. Heat up the oil in a large pot on medium heat. Add in the sofrito/recaito and the crushed fresh garlic. Sauté for 6 minutes. Add in the chicken breast; brown on all sides. Add in the seasoned vegetables and corn, and pour in enough broth to cover. Add in the chicken bouillon, then cook on high until it reaches a boil. Cover, lower heat to medium, and continue to simmer for 3 hours, stirring occasionally. Serve with white rice and sliced avocado, if desired.

Note: This recipe can be made ahead of time and frozen. Just make the rice fresh.

....

Pot Roast

Pot roast is great because of the high amount of protein and iron that you can get from it. It also freezes well and is easy to make because you prep and let it cook on its own for a few hours. This recipe uses bone broth for added nutritional benefits. Make an effort to get organic, grass-fed beef, but if you aren't able to, use what you have access to.

1 bottom round roast

¼ cup white vinegar

2 tablespoons avocado oil

1 tablespoon butter

1 large yellow onion, thinly sliced

2 tablespoons paprika

¼ tablespoon adobo

½ tablespoon garlic powder

¼ tablespoon onion powder

½ tablespoon black pepper

½ tablespoon salt (you can reduce this as needed if you need a lower-sodium version)

A few sprigs fresh thyme

20 ounces beef bone broth

1 (1-pound) bag of baby carrots

6 large yellow potatoes, peeled and cut into chunks

Optional: additional vegetables of your choosing

Rinse the roast with cool water. Trim any large layers of fat that may be on the bottom of the roast. Place in a large bowl and cover with water. Add the vinegar to the bowl and allow to sit for 10 minutes. Meanwhile, preheat the oven to 325 degrees F and thinly slice your onion. Heat the oil over medium heat in a large Dutch oven. Remove the roast from the bowl, rinse, dry, and rub the seasonings except the thyme, all over. Then sear on all sides in the Dutch oven. Remove and set aside on a plate. Add the butter and the onions to the pot. Stir, making sure to scrape up any brown bits with a wooden spoon. Cook the onions down a bit until they're browned and translucent. Deglaze by adding in the beef bone broth, give it a stir, and then add in the roast and thyme. Follow up by adding in the potatoes and carrots. Make sure the potatoes and carrots are immersed in the broth. Put the lid on the pot and place in the oven. Cook for a minimum of 4 hours. If you wish to cook it longer, just keep an eye on it. When it's finished, the meat should fall apart. Serve with egg noodles or rice, or just eat as is.

Gravy

Liquid from roast

¼ cup flour

Optional: salt or seasoned salt, to taste

When the roast is finished, remove everything from the pot except the liquid at the bottom. Place on the stove over medium heat. Add the flour to a mesh strainer and gently tap to add some of it into the liquid, whisking quickly as you do. Continue cooking and gradually adding more of the flour until you reach your desired thickness. You may not need to add all the flour; take your time with this. Do not add more than ¼ cup. If you find that you added too much, add a splash of hot water to thin it out, or any residual beef bone broth you may have in the carton. If you feel called to, feel free to add salt or seasoned salt.

....

HERBAL SUGGESTIONS

- Burn onion and garlic skins on a piece of charcoal to cleanse spaces or yourself of anything funky or the evil eye.

- Place lemons in a bowl to absorb negative energy in the home; replace immediately with new ones if they become moldy. If they simply dry out, toss them in a garbage can outside your home.

- Burn dragon's-blood incense for protection.

- Sprinkle black salt in a line across your doorway for a protective boundary.

- Hang a sachet of dried elderflower above your doorway for protection from hexes.

- Hang a calendula wreath on your front door to prevent negative energy from entering your home.

AFFIRMATIONS

- Each stage of my journey is preparing me for the next.

- I am deserving of a team that supports me fully.

- My wants and needs are a priority.

- Anyone who does not respect my needs does not deserve access to me.

CHAPTER 6

LABOR AND BIRTH

My mom loved to be pregnant and loved the process of giving birth. To this day, she tells everyone she would have done it many times over. Not everyone feels this way, but then again, she is an Aquarius who often finds joy in things many do not (such as coming back to earth time and time again, no matter how hard it is). She is spiritually gifted in her own way, especially when it comes to the spirit of life. I am her firstborn, and every year on my birthday, she shares the story of my birth, her joy radiating. She went into labor in the middle of the night, in the middle of a blizzard, in the tiny Brooklyn apartment she and my dad lived in. She went to the hospital in the morning and had me shortly after. She told me how she stood in the shower, letting the water work its magic, visualizing me moving down the canal, the two of us working as a team. Such a short and easy labor with a first child is typically unheard of. Somehow, though, she—or should I say we—made it happen. She always shares the same details, including the part where my dad drove up a one-way street the wrong way to get to the hospital and how her childhood best friend who drove down for the occasion lost her car keys in the snow and Dad helped her find them.

Something special that my dad shared with me about my birth is that he was so enamored that he went out and bought a ring (my parents were already married) to honor the occasion. He gifted it to my mom, and they gave it to me on my eighteenth birthday. Push-day presents are typically given by a partner, but don't feel shy about doing this for yourself! I bought myself a ring with my child's birthstone that I plan on giving to them on their eighteenth birthday. It's my own way of carrying on the tradition that my parents started. Think about what traditions you want to begin or continue around your baby's birth.

As I was preparing for the birth of my firstborn, my mom shared something important with me: In that first moment of holding your baby, tune everything out. You only have a few seconds, maybe a minute, for this. Home in on your baby, on their energy. Feel who they are. Let it be revealed. Drop all expectations, all hopes, and just receive. Are they sensitive? Are they already a bit more independent than average? Are they an old soul? Do they have an intense energy? Is their energy gentler than most? If you're having a scheduled cesarean, ask your providers about a "gentle C-section"—in which you're still able to hold the baby soon after birth—so that you can have this experience.

My mom says she knew immediately that I was an old, sensitive soul with an intense energy that would require a different kind of support and that I would not take to just anyone. I'm still like this in many ways. When she had my brother, she knew he had a calmer and airier energy, that he was the type who would go where the wind blew him (no surprise, he's a Libra).

This isn't about projecting onto your baby, it's about receiving and taking in who they are at face value, not so you can change them, but so you can know how to support them. When I tuned into my baby, I knew, *Wow, this baby has been here many times before, and remembers, too.* I also knew they were sensitive and gifted in ways that would be revealed with time. It came in like a wave, crashing on the shore of my heart and mind, bringing this sense of knowing to me with ease. As I took in their face, I could see that this was a baby I had birthed in a previous lifetime, one whom I had seen in a past-life regression session with my elder Yvonne Secreto. No wonder they felt so familiar even while in the womb. Now we were reunited once again.

....

A Note About Inducing Labor "Naturally"

Technically anything we do to bring on labor is not natural, even if what is used is. In most cases, your body and the baby work together to decide when is best. However, if you are called to try to bring labor on, here are some safe options: nipple stimulation, sex (ejaculation can help soften your cervix), curb stepping (a walking pattern that can help bring on labor and get baby in the right position: walk with one foot on the curb and another on the street), and bouncing on an exercise ball. Please do not use castor oil, unless you are okay with the runs, which is more likely what you'll end up with.

If you want to find herbal support, ask your midwife or doctor about using evening primrose oil, which worked extremely well for me. If you get the okay, prick a hole in the capsule and insert it vaginally.

There is nothing wrong with doing what you can to induce; you don't have to be the champion of waiting it out. Part of birthing on your terms is doing that in all stages. Always consult your birth team and medical provider before making any intervention.

....

When I was a few days shy of forty weeks, I was ready. I felt like I was having contractions and my chiropractor told me, "Your body is getting ready for labor." The women on my mother's side have a history of babies being born en caul (in the amniotic sac), so I knew not to expect my water to break early. Once it began, my labor lasted for days.

At one point in the evening of day two, as I lay on my side in the bed trying to ride the wave, my mom and partner rubbing my back, the room became filled with a different energy. My spiritual team packed in, including my dad, spirit guides, and other relatives who had passed. It brought me to tears as, one by one, each gave me words of encouragement, affirming that I could do this and was closer than I knew. Telling me about those who did it before me. Reminding me that I was not alone and of the strength not just in me but in them. I cried tears of joy. The warmth I felt from them was soothing and empowering, like a bear hug. I had carried so much grief about my dad not being alive during my pregnancy, never getting to ever hold my baby. But there he was. To feel the strength of them all in the room was everything. I spoke with and cried to them; I thanked them. I felt them soothing me with their energy, reaching out to me. They surrounded me and made it clear that they had a role in ushering this soul into the world. Labor can feel like you're alone, but it was clear that I wasn't alone. (Fortunately, my mom was able to explain to my midwife and doula what was happening, because it looked like I was having a breakdown. Lighting candles and praying at my altar was one thing; this was another entirely.)

When my body finally told me it was time, I was exhausted. This was the third day of labor. It was almost seven in the morning. The sun was coming up. I announced to the room, "I need to push." My team rushed to add more hot water to the birthing pool, but I insisted I just wanted to get in. Something clicked. I sank into the water. I did not resist; I let it flow. I allowed my intuition to guide me. With each contraction, I breathed down deep into my body, visualizing my baby moving along. In between contractions, I tried to relax, doing what I could not to tense up, keeping my face soft, jaw unclenched. I kept hearing, "Release, relax." I moaned deeper and deeper with each release. I felt myself actively bridging the realms so that my baby could cross. It was one of the most otherworldly experiences I have ever had.

The head emerged, and the midwife encouraged me to reach down and feel it. I cradled a full head of hair in my palm. Moments after, my baby shot out into the water, and into the world, like a swimmer in a pool. I scooped them out of the water, held them, and took it all in. Their energy, their face—oh, that beautiful face I had waited so long for. I placed them on my chest as they looked at me with eyes like mine, eyes that said, "Hello again." I felt time stop. Nothing but us even existed. Nothing else mattered.

Intuition plays a key role in labor and birthing. It can let us know when something is wrong, it can let us know when it's time to push, it can let us know how to push. To allow your intuition and body to work together, remember that anxiety creates fear and confusion and is committed to presenting you with all the worst possible scenarios. Intuition brings clarity and is direct. Both are part of the human experience. To some extent, anxiety can keep us safe by occupying our minds with the task of being aware of the possible dangers or threats. Intuition can do this, too, but offers a balanced solution. When you are feeling confused, take a deep breath and remind yourself that anxiety is committed to convincing you the worst is inevitable. Your intuition is committed to guiding and supporting you. While your intuition may let you know that something is wrong, it will help you to take action to address it, not overwhelm you. Anxiety will try to inhibit you from taking action. Be mindful of where you feel anxiety in your body on a daily basis. It's different for everyone. I experience anxiety in my stomach and become nauseated when those nerves kick in. Others experience anxiety in their legs and bounce their leg or tap their foot. When this happens, take a few deep breaths and center yourself. Take back the wheel from anxiety and redirect your thoughts. Like a car on a highway, you can get off at the next exit.

EXERCISE:
CALLING IN YOUR ANCESTORS

Your ancestors and spirits are part of your birth team. You may feel alone at certain moments during labor and birth, but you aren't. The room is filled with anyone who is there to support you in this transitional moment, including those who aren't here in the physical plane. Our ancestors are always with us; they're everywhere. A simple way to call them in if you feel the need to is to state out loud, "I call upon my honorable ancestors to come forth for what is about to take place. I am so thankful for your presence in my life: your many blessings, the protection you bestow upon me, and the way you walk with me. I ask that in this time you bring me strength so that I may give birth safely and timely."

....

How to Personalize the Hospital Experience

If you're birthing in a hospital, so much can feel like it is out of your control. Your birth team will play a key role in supporting and advocating for you, the same way they would at a home birth or a birthing center. Honor your body with decisions about pain management, such as whether to have an epidural. There is nothing wrong with choosing to have one, or any other way to manage pain. We all have unique tolerances and needs. Be attentive to your intuition, especially if you feel a doctor or staff member is not prioritizing your safety or listening to you. Be firm and do not doubt yourself—your doctor is not experiencing your symptoms, you are.

Unfortunately, many hospital staff are overworked and our for-profit healthcare system runs like a business, prioritizing what is most "efficient" rather than focusing on personalized care. While it is, of course, not always the case, it is pretty common for laboring people to sense expediency being emphasized above all. This doesn't mean you have to forgo a hospital birth if that is where you feel safest or if you were medically advised to give birth there. No matter where or how you birth, there is always a possibility that things may not go as you planned or hoped—and there are also things that you can do to be as prepared and comfortable as possible.

Create guidelines with your doula and/or birth team and put them in writing. Post them on the door of your hospital room for the staff to see and refer to. It can help to have an easy reference for your preferences without needing to repeat yourself—or to remember when you're deep in it. It also can make it easier for your partner or doula to advocate for your wants and needs, such as immediate skin-to-skin contact, support and encouragement within the golden hour for breast/bodyfeeding, or what you'd prefer if you need to have an unplanned C-section (such as a gentle C-section). Feel free to look up options online or ask other parents in your community what worked for them. For example, you can request to skip the baby's first bath to preserve the vernix caseosa—the creamy white protective skin coating that baby is born with—and gently rub it in over the first forty-eight hours.

Cleanse the Room

A few weeks before your due date, prepare a cleansing spray from the options below to bring to the hospital, and put it in your go-bag. When you arrive, spray it on the sheets, on the pillow, and around the room.

Blend 1: One part frankincense hydrosol, one part chamomile hydrosol, and one part lavender hydrosol. This is a cleansing and calming blend to help shift the energy and maintain your peace.

Blend 2: One part lemon hydrosol, one part lime hydrosol, one part rosemary hydrosol. This is a purifying blend with an energizing pick-me-up effect. After use, follow up with something sweet, such as rose or lavender hydrosol.

Blend 3: Get a bottle of sandalwood cologne and pour the liquid into a spray bottle. Spray around the room and even on yourself to help you to stay grounded during labor.

Blend 4: Get a bottle of Kolonia 1800 and a bottle of orange blossom water. Mix in equal parts and fill a small spray bottle with the blend. Spray this around the room and on yourself to cleanse, and ease anxiety.

While still at home, call on your ancestors of the highest vibration and light a candle, asking them to ensure a safe delivery and postpartum experience for both you and the baby. Leave an offering on your altar of something sweet that they enjoyed in their lifetime or that is culturally relevant.

Communicate with the higher selves of the hospital staff by visualizing them and speaking to them, asking them to provide you with the best care. You can do this either in the hospital or at home before you go.

....

What If Your Birth Doesn't Go as Planned?

Say you planned to birth at home but needed to be transported to the hospital instead. Or you had an unplanned C-section. While this rearrangement can be disappointing, and even traumatizing, depending on the circumstances, it does not mean you failed. Sometimes, things shift, for so many reasons. Take time to process your emotions, but do your best to keep perspective. This wasn't a reflection of you as a parent or a person. It simply was a matter of chance or variables beyond your control. It could be that you weren't properly supported, someone else was negligent, or your baby had other plans. Sometimes shit just happens. What is in your control is what you do after.

Before you're in the moment, consider your usual response to disappointment or trauma. Do you take time to heal? Do you try to sweep it under the rug? Do you spend time blaming yourself? You decide how you move forward. That is a way of reclaiming your power and narrative, which you are absolutely capable of doing. Work within a time frame that honors your personal capacity. There is no need to rush or follow a timeline of what you think is expected of you.

....

PACKING LIST

Make a batch of oatmeal cookies to support your milk supply and replenish yourself after birth. You can also bring any supplements you're considering taking, such as moringa leaf.

Energetic aids for your hospital or birthing center bag: Bring protective jewelry for the baby and for you, such as an azabache or other charms and energetic sprays or spiritual colognes/waters. This way, you can have your partner or a member of your birth team, such as your doula, sprinkle or spray some throughout the room while praying to cleanse any leftover energies.

If you want to add ambiance or softer lighting, bring electric tea lights or other electric candles. These can also be used in place of traditional candles for prayer or setting intentions.

Bring the swaddles and clothes you washed with rose or chamomile hydrosol, which are infused with loving and calming energy while still being gentle on your little one's skin, to assist them in making a smooth transition to being earth-side.

WHAT ABOUT MY PLACENTA?

You'll need to decide ahead of time what (if anything) to do with the placenta, which is the tissue that connected your baby to your uterus via the umbilical cord and provided all the nutrients they needed for nine months. It is delivered after the baby. Once you've delivered your placenta and are enjoying some more skin-to-skin with baby, you'll receive what is called a fundal massage. This is done to encourage healing of the uterus, helping it to contract and go back to its original size, and prevent postpartum hemorrhaging.

If you want to keep your placenta for any purpose, see below.

For a home birth, you need a large bowl or Tupperware. I would advise choosing a bowl or Tupperware specifically for this use. It's my personal belief that the same way you break out the fine china for special occasions or have a special cake plate you use for birthdays only, the same action should be taken for this bowl or Tupperware. Honor that this is a special event, and let it be dedicated for this use only. It doesn't have to be expensive, but you should still make it special. I used a beautiful, large, gold-colored bowl that cost me less than twenty dollars. You can keep it as a memento, but I would suggest using it specifically for things associated with birth, for this baby or others to come.

If you're birthing at a hospital or birthing center, make your decision known ahead of time and be clear about your choice. I've been told by friends and clients that it was difficult to get the hospital to honor the parents' decision about taking the placenta with them. Try to get it in writing that this is what you'll be doing with your placenta. You should plan to bring a cooler stocked with plenty of ice to keep the placenta cool until your encapsulator arrives or until you are able to bring it home and put it in the fridge.

In some traditions, women consume their placenta after birth, which may help avoid postpartum depression, provide supportive nutrients, and aid in postpartum recovery. Look up "placenta encapsulation"; many doulas have a side hustle in this and can advise. You can also prepare it in a dish, such as stir-fry style, ideally under the watch of someone who is familiar with the practice.

Other traditions involve burying the placenta. I personally see the placenta as the companion of the baby. This companion was essential in the baby's process of coming earth-side, and burying it not only honors the companion but gives the baby a strong connection to the earth. For some it is about connecting the baby to their community or symbolizing that they always have somewhere to return to. Be intentional about where you choose to bury it. Herbs and roots are sometimes buried along with the placenta; which ones vary from person to person and culture to culture, but you can include easily accessible ones, such as angelica root, lavender, rosemary, and rose. Say some prayers for your baby and give thanks to the placenta. When my baby was born, the ground was still frozen, so we stored the placenta in the freezer until the spring thaw. Bury it in a muslin bag and place rocks over the site to avoid animals digging it up.

THE FIRST FORTY DAYS

For the first forty days postpartum, you want to say no to company other than family (as defined by you), friends, or a postpartum doula who is specifically there to help with the baby and allow you to rest. Avoid any unnecessary outings. In some Latin American cultures, this is referred to as your cuarentena, but many other traditional cultures around the world take the same approach.

The purpose of this lying-in period is to support your uterus and body in healing. Ask your loved ones to make sure you don't experience added stress, and eat a lot of broths, soups, stews, and other hearty, nutrient-dense, warm meals to replenish you. Avoid stepping onto cold floors without thick socks and eating too many cold or highly processed foods, and do your best to lie down (with your baby!) for most of the day.

Whether you had a vaginal birth or a C-section, you have a wound in your uterus that is about the size of a dinner plate from the placenta—and if you had a C-section, you also need to tend to your incision. Be gentle with yourself, and do not rush into physical activity or hitting the gym. Otherwise, down the line, your body will remind you of this choice in a variety of unpleasant ways. The one thing you may want to consider doing (but not right away) is finding a pelvic-floor therapist to help you recover from pregnancy and birth. It is different for each individual, but the changes to your pelvic floor can cause incontinence, pain during sex, hip pain, lower back pain, and more. There are symptoms that may not be experienced until further down the line as well, such as vaginal prolapse. Many may be familiar with Kegels, which are about tightening and releasing the muscles in your pelvic floor. This is not the only exercise you can do for your pelvic floor, and it may not be the one best suited to your needs. Take some time to do your research and look into beginning a pelvic-floor therapy practice after your first forty days have passed, allowing a professional to support you.

Press a warm, wet washcloth against your perineum during bowel movements. It makes it easier by reducing pain and fear so you have less anxiety about tearing.

If you have stitches from tearing, apply a high-grade manuka honey daily. This will help with healing and reduce the likelihood of having scar tissue after. If you do scar, you can break it up a bit by using your thumb to gently stretch the tissue after the stitches have dissolved. Sex can also move it around, but beginning with your thumb and having control over the pressure can be a more comfortable experience. It will also reconnect you to your body on a physical and sexual level. This can be particularly helpful if you experienced any birth-related trauma, because it puts you back in control and allows you to do things at your own pace while giving you the room to be present if something comes up that triggers a response.

Your partner may be excited to have sex again, and you may be looking forward to it, too—just keep in mind that the focus of this time is healing. Many people decide to jump back in before the end of the forty days, and that is your decision to make (just consult with your midwife or OB first). But do not allow anyone to pressure you, even into other sexual acts. If you feel that you need more time, take it. Another option is to take the opportunity to connect with your postpartum body, as exploring through self-pleasure—whether clitoral or other external stimulation (such as touching other parts of your body and becoming more familiar with how they've changed as well)—can be a gentler yet still fulfilling approach.

RECLAIMING CHILDBIRTH

Note that you can change your team at any time during your pregnancy, even if it's in the middle of labor. I changed my team and care provider when I hit my third trimester. Who you start with may not be who you finish with. There is no shame in this. You must prioritize your safety, the baby's safety, and the sacredness of your experience. Take note if your team does not support your having a birth plan (of course, plans can change, but you should be supported in having one), if you are pressured into things you don't feel right about or trust, and especially if you feel that racism, discrimination, or implicit bias is a factor in your treatment. Your team should make you feel supported, safe, and trusting that they have your best interest at heart.

Pregnancy and birth can be dangerous. This is why, in many cultures, childbirth is viewed as a battle, one that the warrior must be prepared for and supported through, with their wounds tended to and their battle scars honored. In the United States, childbirth is exceptionally dangerous for Black women, whose concerns and pain are too often dismissed by medical teams. Brown women experience much of the same at lower rates. There are many ways the injustice of medical racism plays out, and while injury and death are possibilities for anyone giving birth, let's not shy away from the differences in how, why, and the frequency at which they occur, which can help individuals to shape a proper birth team and plan. On a larger scale, it can help us implement the systemic changes that would make birthing a more equitable experience for all. It's critical that access to care providers who prioritize both safety and autonomy is available to everyone. Unfortunately, nothing and no one can protect you from every contingency. But we can do our best to try.

Birthing safely and on your terms is an act of decolonization and resistance for everyone. While childbirth has always carried the risks of death and complications, living in a colonized society causes these risks to increase for a variety of reasons, including implicit bias, medical racism, and the industrialization of birth. Consider the women of Puerto Rico who were sterilized without their knowledge and consent, as well as those who became the test subjects for modern-day birth control (leading to infertility for many), and the

Black maternal health crisis that is still ongoing. To do what the systems put in place are trying to prevent you from doing is an act of resistance.

It is an opportunity for ancestral healing as well— an opportunity to reconnect with the ways your ancestors birthed, to heal those who came before you whose cries for help were dismissed. To heal those who experienced violence in their birthing experience, to heal those who came earth-side in a violent manner (with the use of forceps and other tools that have largely fallen out of use).

You have an opportunity to do this, and you are deserving of seizing that opportunity. If not for you, then for those who came before you and those who are going to come from you. Remember: you are not "difficult" because you want quality care, plain and simple.

HERBAL SUGGESTIONS

- **Evening primrose oil to help with dilation:**
  With your provider's agreement, prick a capsule and insert vaginally.

- **Frankincense to cleanse and bless the space:**
  Burn on a charcoal tablet to smoke-cleanse or spray a frankincense hydrosol.

AFFIRMATIONS

- I am deserving of a birthing experience that I want to remember.

- My concerns are valid and are to be respected.

- I am a human, not a machine in a factory; my birthing experience will be unique to me.

- I have faith in my birthing team.

CHAPTER 7

MISCARRIAGE, STILLBIRTHS, AND RAINBOW BABIES

F eel free to skip this chapter if this topic feels triggering, traumatic, taboo, or stressful for you. Please note that any suggestions can also be useful in the aftermath of stillbirths.

Miscarriage is far more common than most people know, especially in the first twelve weeks of pregnancy, often making that a both joyful and stressful time of waiting. (It can occur at any stage, but it's less likely after the first trimester, which is why health practitioners often advise waiting until then to share the news.) Recently, the term "rainbow babies" has become more popular and publicly used. Rainbow babies are birthed after a previous miscarriage—because after the storm comes a rainbow.

A few years ago, my child's father and I were trying to conceive. I felt it in my heart and spirit that a baby wanted to come into this world through us. My ancestors and guides had made it clear. I kept seeing signs everywhere. During a full-moon event at a friend's yoga studio, the baby's spirit was presented to me. We were in meditation, after drinking blue lotus tea (it was a blue moon), when I had a profound experience with this baby's spirit. Several of my ancestors extended their hands out toward me. They were holding a beautiful baby, her eyes like mine, sparkling. A glowing iridescent light surrounded her. I felt so much warmth coming over me, it was as though the energy itself was hugging me. I cried tears of joy as my ancestors told me that this was the baby coming to me. That her spirit was coming to me, in her time. To be patient, as things were happening with divine timing. Later that evening, I shared with my partner what I had experienced, and he, too, was filled with joy. We continued to be intentional with our efforts to conceive, and come summer, I had a positive pregnancy test, which I had taken after feeling a shift in my body—I could tell that I was no longer alone. There were two of us. A sweet, bright, and loving spirit was within me. I was elated, but it was still early. I shared the news only with my partner, my mom, and two close friends. Keeping it close to my heart was my first act of protection for this blessing. My partner had to go out of town for work and would be gone for the summer. I spent my days talking to the baby, rubbing my pelvis, seeing my friends, thanking my ancestors, and getting excited, and I began taking prenatal vitamins and looking for baby clothes.

One day, I woke up with an excruciating pain beyond any cramps I had ever had. I immediately knew that something was wrong. I called my mom, who suggested I do my best to relax. I got into a warm bath and wrote to a doula friend, who advised me to drink ginger tea. But I knew it was already too late. I could feel this baby's spirit leaving. A few minutes after getting out of the bath, I felt an intense wave of pain and saw the blood. I felt compelled to push. I was miscarrying. I felt my heart break in a way I had never known it could.

I had experienced the death of people close to me, including my dad's a few years before. Like every death, this one was different. I could not understand what had happened and why. I cried in bed for hours and chose not to tell my child's father, who was in another state at the time and needed to focus on work. I also knew that he wouldn't be able to support me at a distance the way I needed in that moment.

That night I had a dream in which the explanation came to me. I already knew that I was not the first in my family to experience this kind of loss, and I wouldn't be the last. The miscarriage wasn't a reflection of my ability or worthiness to become a mother—which is true for everyone who has experienced miscarriage. I woke feeling the vision's healing and understanding inside of me. While this didn't make everything "better," it did give me a sense of closure, which, after all, is something we need to make ourselves.

We continued to try to conceive, and now I knew that I would birth a baby, in time. The following year I entered what is referred to in astrology as my Saturn return, which is when Saturn is in the same sign as when you were born and remains there for two and a half years. I booked a reading with an astrologist to gain her insight. I had been feeling the shift in energy already, and messages from my guides and ancestors made it clear that another baby (and much more) was coming. From work life to my relationship, there was a lot transforming, she told me. Then she mentioned a pregnancy that summer. I couldn't help but smile; it was written in the stars. I felt more hopeful than I had in a long time—since my miscarriage.

In the beginning of the summer, I felt that shift in my body once again. It was no longer just me there. I had asked my spirits not to present me with the spirit, as they had before, but to simply let me experience it this time. I needed to experience it differently. As every baby is different, I wanted that to be honored from the start. This spirit felt strong and fiery yet sweet. It also felt like one I had known before, but not in this lifetime. I kept the news to myself and waited to share it with anyone, including my child's father. This was a sacred moment that I wanted to indulge in. I spent time talking with the baby, encouraging the baby to get comfortable—we were in it for the long haul this time.

At the end of July, I felt a discomfort in my womb and became concerned. It was about six in the morning, and I insisted my child's father take me to the hospital. This was still the first year of the COVID-19 pandemic, so he wasn't allowed to come in. Once again, I was alone. While at first the hospital staff insisted it was probably nothing, they finally agreed to look into it. I gave a urine sample and they arranged a vaginal ultrasound. During the ultrasound, I felt as though my hand was being held by my dad. I heard a whisper of his voice saying, "Congratulations, my sweetie," and that everything was going to be fine, that I'd soon be able to share the news.

Shortly after, they came in and confirmed I was about five weeks pregnant. My womb was simply expanding to make room for the baby, and the discomfort was nothing to be worried about. I knew, but now I could share it with my loved ones.

My pregnancy was intentional on every front. I took nothing for granted. I worked with elders and checked in regularly to see if there was anything I needed to do. I talked to my baby, even before they could hear my voice. I prayed multiple times a day. For me, this was important because I was not only praying but communicating with my baby's spirit.

One night during the first trimester, my baby's spirit came to me in a dream and told me their name.

My labor was long (days long), and my ancestors, as well as the baby I had miscarried, were present for all of it. The privilege of holding my rainbow baby, skin to skin, feeling that physical reconnection, will remain with me forever.

As my baby has grown, I've had moments in which I wish that their sibling were here. I know, though, that that first baby was essential in this baby's arrival—assisting in guiding in the spiritual plane, encouraging in a way only siblings can. I hold my baby a bit tighter when the anniversary of my miscarriage comes each year, the same way I rubbed my pregnant belly more often that first time around.

The sadness and feeling of missing aren't gone. I don't believe they ever will be. Even if my first baby and I are reunited in this lifetime, I know I'll still feel sad that it took that long for us to come back together. What has changed, though, is how I interact with the experience—not because I had a baby, but because I changed the nature of our relationship. I still talk to her, I still light a candle for her, I still think of her. I still pray she will come back around. A few espiritistas/spiritualists I know have said that she will, and I know in my heart that this is true, but I try to hold it loosely. Time has given me the room to understand and accept that wasn't an ending for us but a redirection. Not everyone will feel the same, and that's okay. We all grieve and process differently. We all have different perspectives. There is no right or wrong.

Healing from a miscarriage or miscarriages will not look the same for everyone. Womb work (such as healing ceremonies for the womb and womb massage) or energy work (such as Reiki) can be powerful, especially if you work with a practitioner so you can be supported fully. We often experience miscarriages alone and suffer in silence, and we shouldn't have to with our healing, too. A facilitator can hold space and take action in a way that supports your ability to heal yourself. We all need that kind of support because we are communal beings. Part of that means accepting your community's role of helping you when you need it.

PRACTICES TO
HONOR AND HEAL

If you'd like to set up a small altar space to pray at and light candles for the baby's spirit, honor that. Start by cleansing the space with frankincense and wiping down the surface with Florida water. Place a white cloth down, along with a glass of water, a white candle, an ultrasound photo if you have one, and perhaps a small toy. Pray for the baby's spirit to be elevated and let them know how loved they are. This can be a place for you to mourn.

Another option is to go to a church and dedicate a mass to that baby. If this is part of your spiritual practice or tradition, or you'd like it to be, you can attend mass and dedicate all your prayers said during the service to the baby, either out loud or in your heart. You can also give the name of the baby to the priest or simply say "Child of [your name]" so that everyone in attendance dedicates their prayer to uplifting the baby's spirit. The purpose is to have all those prayers and energy dedicated to supporting that baby's spirit in their transition. You can also put together a prayer circle with people close to you instead.

Some say that the baby you have after a miscarriage is the spirit returned, but this is not always true. There are many reasons that miscarriages happen, physically and spiritually. The spirit does not always return in your next pregnancy, or even in this lifetime. There are many possibilities related to both the baby's path and your own. For example, it may have been in that baby's path to awaken you to the reality that you want children or to kindle a kind of love you never experienced before. This doesn't mean you did anything wrong. There is so much that we don't have control over, in both life and death. Surrendering can be the most difficult part of healing, pregnancy, labor, and loss. You are capable, though, and it is a journey, not a race.

If you are curious to explore where your baby comes from, there are a few things that can help you to decipher whether this baby is one that has returned from a previous miscarriage. You've probably heard of a mother's intuition, which doesn't always kick in right away; it can develop its strength and presence over time. Sit in meditation and ask about your baby. There may already be a sense of knowing. Or you can go the route of letting the child and their spirit show you as time goes on. Children will always tell you who they are; it's up to us to be open enough to hear them when they do.

You can work with different forms of divination, such as tarot or Akashic records readings, or seek spiritual counsel from other diviners as well. There are many kinds of readings or divinations you can receive, and how they are performed will vary. You may need what is referred to as a spiritual mass for your healing and to help elevate the baby's spirit. This may be something that is brought up in your reading as well. Typically, a practitioner will use their tools or method of choice to relay the information to you.

HERBAL SUGGESTIONS

- Chamomile infusion for soothing nerves and support with anxiety. Add a cinnamon stick before steeping with boiling water to warm the body and aid with healing.

- Speak with an herbalist about working with rue to cleanse and heal the womb. There are other options, such as stinging nettle, but rue in particular helps to cleanse by stimulating uterine contractions.

AFFIRMATIONS

- A loss is a loss, no matter how early, and so I honor my heart's grief fully.

- The love I have for my baby transcends all planes and protects them in every realm.

- My timeline may feel difficult and unkind, but like the ocean, there will inevitably be a change in the tide.

CHAPTER 8

FOURTH TRIMESTER

The fourth trimester—or those hectic and precious months after the baby is born—is no less important than the first, second, or third. Healing from birth is complicated, and so is adjusting to life with a newborn. You'll hear, "Sleep when the baby sleeps," but what if you need to clean the house when the baby sleeps? What if you need to cook when the baby sleeps? What if your baby will only sleep on you? It can be overwhelming (even more so if you have another kid).

MENTAL HEALTH: PPD, PPA, PPP

Mental health becomes its own challenge, and not just because of sleep deprivation. Postpartum depression, postpartum anxiety, and postpartum psychosis are real, so please seek out professional support if you are experiencing any symptoms, which are not limited to but can include hallucinations, delusions, mania, mood swings, feelings of hopelessness, withdrawing from family and friends, changes in appetite, insomnia or oversleeping, loss of interest in things you enjoy, intense irritability and anger, feelings of shame or worthlessness, reduced ability to think clearly and make decisions, thoughts of harming yourself or your baby, overwhelming anxiety, paranoia, and suicidal thoughts.

None of these should be written off as a result of not being prepared, not being accepting of parenthood, or any other explanation that doesn't involve a deeper look. While these can exacerbate things, it's crucial not to claim that they're the sole cause without further investigation. The postpartum drop in hormones is intense on the body and has a direct impact on mental health. There are many options for treatment that are not limited to medication (though there is no shame in taking medication). You don't have to suffer in silence or just try to change your mindset. There is a reason so many traditional practices are centered around supporting a new parent. Don't deprive yourself of support; your ancestors would want you to receive it.

After we give birth, our gray brain matter shrinks, and this can last for two years following your most recent birth. Our brain literally changes not only during pregnancy but upon giving birth. Combine this with a hormonal drop, and it's a perfect storm that can leave you feeling like you are an entirely different person.

It is unrealistic for people to expect you to "be yourself again" shortly after giving birth. It's also unrealistic for you to expect this of yourself, especially because you won't be yourself again. You'll be a new version of yourself. (More on that later.) Many birth workers share the phrase "postpartum is forever" because the impact of having children on your body, mind, and soul lasts a lifetime.

While your gray matter may shift again down the line, it doesn't mean you can't have postpartum depression or postpartum anxiety simply because the six-month mark has passed. Weaning (at any age) can cause a flare-up in mental health issues more frequently than people realize.

Take your time; don't be hard on yourself if you are more forgetful than usual or if you find yourself feeling like someone in *Invasion of the Body Snatchers*. There is far more going on than what meets the eye. While it would be nice if there were a simple ritual to pass through this time with as much grace for yourself as possible, the real ritual is community support and care. The ritual is to try a little tenderness for yourself. There's only so much you can do to counteract and remedy the hormonal roller coaster, so you have to ride it as best you can.

INTEGRATING YOUR
NEW IDENTITY

The fourth trimester was relatively easy for me and baby; reconnecting with myself was not so easy. I was isolated because of the pandemic. I didn't see much of other adults, during both my pregnancy and postpartum. It took a toll. While we hear about motherhood being isolating, we also hear of the sense of community it brings: the opportunity to go to a breastfeeding group or mommy-and-me yoga class. I didn't get to experience any of this. I loved being with my baby day in and day out, but I was missing time with my homegirls and the outside world. I was missing my sense of self. I excelled at being a mom, but in many ways, I was failing at being a person. I knew who I was as a mom, but I had no idea who I was as a person, as a woman, anymore. It made for a rocky time in my life in some areas, while I felt grounded in others.

I still find myself years later making an effort to build a relationship with who I am and to come to know who I'm going to be. While no one can tell you how to do this, what I can say is: You can't go back to who you were.

You can only go forward. As hard as that is, especially considering it's much like a second puberty (yuck!), there is beauty in the opportunity to reinvent ourselves. To evolve beyond the version of ourselves we created. Consider yourself to be a world-class artist who is now in a new stage of their creative career. The world is waiting to see what you'll put forth. You can wow them, and yourself, if you give yourself the room to.

One of my favorite ways to have people connect with themselves during a period of reinvention, or getting to know themselves again, is mirror work: each day for at least twenty-eight days, you speak affirmations or even just words of kindness to yourself in the mirror. It's simple but effective. Your brain begins to create new thought pathways, and you begin to associate yourself with these words of kindness/affirmations. Speaking to yourself in the mirror isn't always comfortable at first, but it helps your brain to see you as you speak words of positivity and encouragement. It learns to associate your self-image with those words.

To remember to make mirror work a regular practice, write reminders on sticky notes and put them on mirrors throughout your home. This way, you can take a beat each time you pass one.

Take the self-love up a notch by anointing yourself with rose oil. This is safe even if you are nursing.

BIRTH TRAUMA

If you experienced birth trauma, that can add another layer of stress in the postpartum period. If there is anything about your birth that isn't sitting right, don't dismiss that instinct. Seek out support in the form of a therapist or healer. Speak about it with other moms or parents in your life; you might be surprised at how many have had similar experiences. Community can be healing. Knowing that you aren't alone and are surrounded by empathetic people is powerful. They can be a sounding board for you to bounce things off. Suffering in silence harms us. Talking brings clarity. When you get it off your chest and out of your head, it makes it easier to breathe again.

Working with elders in your life can be medicine as well. Go to those who can hold space for you. They possess so much wisdom and healing. Sit at their feet and let them share it with you.

A womb-healing practice: Giving yourself a womb massage can help move out the energetic trauma that resides in that space. Gently massage counterclockwise in a circular motion while visualizing anything negative, stagnant, or traumatic leaving your womb. Then go clockwise while visualizing a green healing energy filling your womb. Do this for a few minutes each day; you'll feel the difference. Consider looking into the work of Pānquetzani (@indigemama on Instagram), who shares a practice called the abdominal spiral, a massage technique you can do on yourself.

BODY IMAGE

Body image challenges post-birth are not easy, especially in our snapback culture. They can manifest as feeling like a stranger in your own body or comparing your body to what you see on social media.

I am no stranger to how people can project onto us and be hurtful in that recovery process. Two months postpartum, a family member from my child's father's side commented on my stomach and grabbed it—twice—while asking, "What's going on here?" I did my best to ride the waves of my hormones by extending grace to myself, keeping a journal, and crying when the tears came. Directing my focus to healing, not weight loss, led me to eat whole foods, stews, and nutrient-dense meals. (Besides, the shelf my stomach made was helpful with holding my baby, who gained weight with ease, which is a blessing.) Remind yourself that this is very much like a second puberty. Much of it will more than likely be uncomfortable and feel destabilizing. Your body is adjusting, much like you are. It likely will distribute weight in a way that is beneficial for carrying your baby around on one hip or on your front.

Breast/bodyfeeding won't necessarily make the pounds drop, although everyone says it does; it may instead cause your body to hold on to fat to make milk. On the other hand, you may all of a sudden go from bootylicious to having no booty because your body used up its fat stores there. Our bodies don't follow the trends, though it would be nice if they did. You may be like me—I went from a B cup to a DD, and my hips, thighs, arms, booty—everything—grew alongside.

I cannot stress how important it is to be gentle with yourself and remember it took nine months of your body changing to accommodate a baby, including re-arranging your dang organs. How it continues to change will be as unique as your pregnancy and birth. Remind yourself that unlike those celebs you follow on social media, you don't have an in-home chef, trainer, and plastic surgeon on call.

TOOLS FOR HEALING

- The Magical Faja: One technique I found useful was wearing a faja, which is typically used as shapewear or post-surgery. A faja supports your body in healing by assisting your organs in returning to where they need to be and helping your tummy muscles knit back together (which can prevent diastasis recti, the separation of your abdominal muscles to make room for the growing baby). If you are using a traditional binding garment, such as a rebozo, typically a midwife or birth worker would wrap you, but off-the-shelf shapewear garments, a belly band, or even a stretchy scarf works, too.

- Sitz baths will help heal your perineum and vagina and reduce your hemorrhoids, if you are one of the lucky majority who get them. Pick one up at any drugstore and fill it with hot water and Epsom salt, or even sea salt. Sit in it for fifteen to twenty minutes twice a day. You can also make herbal infusions to add to the bath; consult your birth workers or an herbalist about what they recommend for you, but common herbs for this purpose are plantain leaf, yarrow, calendula, comfrey, lavender, rose, sage, and witch hazel.

- Massaging your womb can expel any stagnant blood and tissue. Do this gently in a clockwise circle or ask your postpartum doula to do it.

- After you are out of the first forty days, consider lymphatic drainage massage, which is a gentle massage that works with your lymphatic system to aid in proper drainage of fluid in the body.

BREAST/BODYFEEDING

Breastfeeding came naturally to me, and baby, which was a blessing. I did work at it, though. I kept my supply up with oats, black seed oil, and supplements, such as moringa. I did a lot of baby wearing and kept my baby close to me. I made sure I ate enough and stayed hydrated.

I did get mastitis a few times until I learned that taking sunflower lecithin can alleviate and prevent it; I didn't get it again, thank goddess. I also used hot compresses to massage my breasts, massaged/hand-expressed in the shower, and used a Haakaa (a type of hand pump that uses suction and can collect milk during letdown) to unclog the ducts by adding warm water and a tablespoon of Epsom salt to it before suctioning it on. The gentle pressure from the suction moved things along. Sometimes I made chamomile tea, poured it into a glass or ceramic bowl, and stuck my whole titty in. You may have heard of using cabbage leaves on an infected breast, but approach this trick with caution because it can dry up your supply (which, if that's your goal, here's a tip on how to do that). Some folks prefer to use cold compresses instead of warm. Find what works for you.

As your body adjusts to breastfeeding, your nipples in particular might feel like they've taken a beating. (And if they are cracked or bleeding, you should consult a lactation consultant; you don't need to live in extreme pain to nurse.) Nipple butter, which is often made of a food-safe oil, such as olive oil or beeswax, and skin-soothing herbs, such as calendula, are commonly used, too, but you might not want to add more moisture into the mix. I preferred witch hazel and would apply it after nursing. It was soothing but still allowed my skin a chance to dry. I recommend saving the nipple butter for after your skin has adjusted a bit.

What was and still is so special to me about body/ breastfeeding is how our bodies connected. Kissing my baby's face helped my body perfectly tailor the antibodies and nutrients in my breast milk. The emptier your breasts/chest, the higher the fat content of your milk, which is why when nursing an infant frequently, you'll find the fat content is higher than if you're still occasionally nursing your toddler. As my baby grew older, my breast milk transformed again to suit their needs, which is why the World Health Organization now recommends breastfeeding for at least two years. Obviously, this is not possible for everyone for a variety of reasons, but I like that that goalpost emphasizes the value in longevity of nursing.

I know that in today's modern world we want to do it all—and I agree that we can and should if we feel called to. That being said, when it comes to breast/bodyfeeding, we don't have to do it all, all at once. Multitasking with hands-free pumps that sit in your bra while you clean or are on the go may be all the rage now, and I respect anyone's desire to use them. But I want to remind you that you can still do it all and not do it all, all at once. Dedicated time that is set aside for pumping is an opportunity for you to take a moment from the other things that life is asking of you. It is a whole-ass job to be a source of sustenance for a baby (or more if you have multiples). Give yourself a break and take some time to pump, catch your breath, and decompress the best you can.

All that said, when it comes to breast/bodyfeeding, formula feeding, or combo feeding, it's a personal choice. Or it may not be a choice at all if your milk didn't come in or you've had a mastectomy or you have to go back to work and are not being properly supported. The same goes for how long you nurse if you do. Do what is best for you and your family.

SETTING BOUNDARIES— EVEN WITH FAMILY

When a baby arrives, people tend to choose to show their ass (to put it bluntly) and give you hell. Sometimes it's with the best of intentions, but not always. This is the last thing you need while recovering, helping your baby adjust to being earth-side, and wrapping your mind around your new life. When a birthing parent isn't supported properly, the fourth trimester will be more difficult than it has to be.

While you were pregnant, you might have felt cared for, but that often stops once the baby has arrived. This isn't an old tradition; it's a new one that doesn't benefit anyone. The traditions of communal support have been forgotten in the U.S. (Other places around the world fortunately have maintained those old traditions of support.) Those who had children helped the new parents learn the ways. Those who did not helped in other ways, from caring for children, to making meals, to healing work. The concept of "it takes a village" honors the varied roles that community fills when children are being raised. In many traditions, that community or village is family. But as we all know, family can sometimes make things worse, whether it's from being overbearing or being critical. This is why boundaries are important, but so is deciding who makes up your village. Choosing not to have certain family members be part of your village is complicated because of our feelings, our connections, our hopes, and societal pressure. No one is entitled to be a part of your inner circle; that is a role that must be earned. Think of it like this: if they don't show up for you in a way that honors and respects you, they won't show up in a way that honors and respects your child, either.

Set boundaries and be firm. Remind everyone that this is your child and your experience. They can do things their way with their family, but you are under no obligation to let them run your show. Turn your broom upside down to get them to leave your home if they're doing too much.

INNER-CHILD HEALING

Inner-child healing is an essential part of the parenting experience. Having children will open you up in ways you did not anticipate, revealing things you need to heal—and they often keep coming. Look at this as an invitation to continue the work, for both you and them. Often people speak of not repeating cycles or doing what their parents did. One way to do that is with boundaries. We can protect our children and heal our inner child this way. Advocating for ourselves goes hand in hand with advocating for our children. It shows them how to one day advocate for themselves and have a true sense of security. Sometimes the way we end a cycle is by cutting ties with those who repeat them. So much of my own healing was about doing just that—saying goodbye to certain family members and keeping at bay anyone who crossed the line, said something out-of-pocket, or was abusive or harmful in any capacity (emotionally, psychologically, verbally, physically). This act of healing provided me and my baby with protection on an energetic and emotional level. Your peace is sacred and something you need to guard, especially in a time of such deep vulnerability. Make no apologies for doing that.

There are many approaches to inner-child healing. Session work is one approach, where you can regress to a childhood memory and facilitate healing around that specific memory.

You can engage in creative activities just for the sake of being creative, with no rules or restrictions—if you're using a coloring book, use whatever colors you want. They don't have to be "correct." Try having play-time or reconnecting with things you loved as a child. My one suggestion would be to pick a simple coloring book if your inner child is having a hard time—the very intricate adult coloring books can exacerbate that.

Reparenting yourself may look like not letting your-self hang out with people who bully you or speaking up to a bully in your life. It may look like creating struc-ture and routine in your life in ways you didn't have growing up.

Choose a picture of yourself as a child and talk to her on a daily basis, with words of encouragement and love. Snuggle with a stuffed animal and visualize yourself hugging your inner child/younger self. Write a letter to your younger self or keep a journal for this pur-pose. With time, you can eventually respond to those letters from the voice and view of your inner child.

Allow yourself to dress colorfully or in a way that you would have wanted to as a child but felt too embar-rassed to or weren't allowed to.

It isn't all ice cream for dinner the way you may have wished as a kid (although there are exceptions while pregnant), but there are many ways to be proactive with this work. Remember, your inner child represents your core wants and needs. So take a deeper look into what they are and how the adult you can take care of them.

DO'S AND DON'TS

Below are some do's and don'ts that have been shared with me over the years. Some of these are superstitions, some are beliefs learned through experience. I don't personally subscribe to each one, but I believe sharing them and considering them can help us be prepared for when our mother-in-law or someone else tries to give us their two cents. As with anything, take what you need and leave what you don't.

Do not set up the crib early to avoid the baby coming too early.

Do not dress your baby in black at night, to protect them from evil spirits. Babies are closer to the spirit realm and thus more susceptible. Choose white or light-colored clothes for bedtime; these colors are reflective of energy rather than absorbent.

Do dress your baby in light colors as often as possible to avoid heavy energies weighing on them. Lighter colors reflect while darker colors absorb; both can be protective, but some colors can be more energetically dense than others because they absorb energy. It's just a different way of working the same ability to be protective.

Do add your milk (if possible) to your baby's baths for protection from energetic harm.

Do not cut your baby's hair until they are at least two years of age to avoid negatively impacting their speech. It should be noted that this is a very old-school and cultural practice, and while there are many factors that can impact speech in children, this is mainly done to avoid exacerbating any preexisting factors at play.

Do save their hair after any and all haircuts so it can be disposed of by you, and make sure no one has access to it to use it for workings against your child. Burn it if possible. The same goes for nail trimmings.

Do not let just anyone do your baby's hair to avoid negative energetic transfer and possible hair loss. Additionally, do not let someone in a bad mood do their hair.

Do not let people who are unkind to you or dislike you hold your baby. It doesn't matter if that's your mother-in-law; your baby doesn't need that energy being transferred to them. They are an extension of you.

Do pull a red string across a baby's forehead to stop hiccups.

Do run warm water over the crown of their head if they are overly fussy (and not sick) to remind them of the womb and move any stagnant energy, especially at night.

Do pat their butt rhythmically to settle them by reminding them of your heartbeat.

Do sprinkle their head and rinse their feet with holy water for blessings and protection.

Do use protective jewelry, such as an azabache or evil eye jewelry.

Do cleanse their space regularly.

Do cleanse them upon leaving the hospital.

Do not take them to the cemetery.

Do your best to avoid taking them out of the home at night (to protect them from wandering spirits).

HERBAL SUGGESTIONS

- In consultation with your birth team, consider nettles in tea form to nourish you and support your recovery, and moringa and black seed oil in capsule form to boost milk supply.

AFFIRMATIONS

- My body is more powerful than I can even imagine; it deserves to be supported.

- I do not need to snap back; I am not a rubber band, I am a human.

- My baby is not the only one new to this role. I am, too, and we're learning together.

CHAPTER 9

BATHS AND SOAKS FOR YOU AND BABY

H erbal baths can be a helpful tool for balancing and shifting energies. We'll go through which herbs are safe to use in baths during pregnancy, while breastfeeding, and/or for a baby.

There are a few ways to prepare an herbal bath. You can pour boiling water over any dry, leafy, or floral herb to steep it, then strain it and allow it to cool before pouring the water over your head/down your body while standing in the bath or shower. (Though traditionally in many practices, cold or room-temperature water is used in the preparation of baths, especially with fresh herbs, you can make a choice.) I prefer using fresh herbs, but they're not always accessible. That's okay! When using hard, dry spices, such as cinnamon sticks or roots, boil for 5 to 15 minutes, strain, and allow to cool before use. Note that various practitioners do baths differently or have other blends they would use or prefer. The differences aren't right or wrong, only different.

During pregnancy and the postpartum period, allow yourself to air-dry after an herbal bath. If it's cold outside, I have often made this easier by keeping a little fan space heater in the bathroom. When getting out of the bath or shower, step onto a mat instead of the cold floor to preserve your womb health and avoid sickness.

When preparing baths for babies, always add the infusion to warm water. If it's warm in the house, allow the baby to air-dry (no air-conditioning!). If the weather and/or your home is cold, gently pat them with a towel. Do not rub.

A soak is different and provides its own physical, as well as energetic, benefits. With a soak, you take that infusion and pour it into your bath, and then, well, you soak in it.

Please take care to ensure that the flowers and herbs used are organic and not grown roadside or with harmful pesticides.

THE BATHS

White Bath

This bath has many variations but the base is generally the same. Use for cleansing your energies and when you need calming or cooling support. Safe for you and your baby.

A white candle in a candleholder with a handle, or a white seven-day candle

1 (13.5-ounce) can coconut milk

Splash of coconut water

1 quart goat milk

1 quart cow's milk

1 teaspoon honey

Sprinkle of cascarilla*

Splash of Florida water or holy water

Sprinkle of cocoa butter

12 white carnations or other white flowers

Cascarilla is powdered eggshell, sometimes mixed with holy water. Make by drying white eggshells in the oven at 325 degrees F for an hour, then blending in a spice blender. You can also buy it at a botanica.

Place the candle in its holder or the seven-day candle in the center of a basin. Add all ingredients to your basin, mix with your hands, and light the candle. Pour water into the basin, using enough to fill a third of your sink or baby tub. Make sure it's hot if preparing it for a baby and cold if preparing it for yourself. Allow the mixture to steep for 20 minutes. Pray over the mixture, asking for cleansing, balancing, protection, a cool mind, peace, and tranquility for your baby (or you). Strain when you feel it's ready. To use for yourself, pour the mixture over yourself while standing in an empty tub or shower, and air-dry. To use for your baby, put them in a sink or empty baby bath, use a sponge to soak the mixture up (making sure it is warm but not hot), and squeeze it over their head as you tilt it back (to avoid getting it in their eyes or mouth), or gently pour it over their body. You can do this for older children as well. Do not rinse. You can pat them dry.

Repeat for three days, or up to nine days. Use your discernment—you can just start with once if that feels right.

Notes: If you have anxiety about honey and botulism occurring if they then put their hands in their mouths after, feel free to wash their hands. Postpartum anxiety is very real, and there is no need to exacerbate it.

Traditionally, after drying from this bath, you would avoid wearing dark colors (wear white, preferably), wrap your head to sleep, and do not have sex, drink, or smoke for the day(s) that you're repeating it. Like we learned in science class, white reflects the sun, while darker colors absorb it. Absorbing energies can be a form of protection, but here we want to avoid any energy weighing you down. Some practitioners say that your sheets should be white as well; this is optional.

....

Rosemary, Basil, Bay Laurel, or Sage Bath

This bath is helpful with general energetic cleansing. Swap the sage for "common" rue (not to be confused with goat's rue) or hyssop when you're not pregnant/nursing for the traditional formulary.

A few fresh bundles of 3 of the 4 herbs, all of which can be bought at the grocery store

Splash of Florida water or holy water

A white candle

Break up the herb bundles by hand in a basin of cold water, praying for the removal of the evil eye/mal de ojo and any heavy, dense, or stagnant energies. Add the Florida water or holy water. Light a white candle in the center of the basin. Continue to pray and speak intention into the bath. When you feel it's complete, remove the candle, strain, and either add to warm water for the baby or pour over yourself while standing in the shower (water off).

This is baby-safe. If you cannot get fresh bay leaves, use fresh sage, and vice versa. You must use three out of what is suggested, such as rosemary, sage, and basil, or bay laurel, basil, and rosemary.

....

Chamomile Bath

This bath is purifying and protective. On a physical level, it is wonderful for teething, colic, and restlessness. You can add equal parts rose and lavender for extra protection and for a boost of unconditional loving energy to comfort baby (although do not add if using this to soak a washcloth in for a teething remedy).

1 tablespoon to 1 cup dried chamomile (see instructions for quantity)

If preparing for an adult, fill a large tea ball with about ½ cup to 1 cup chamomile. Boil 4 to 6 cups of water, pour over tea ball, and steep for 5 to 10 minutes. Allow to cool, and pour over your head and body.

If preparing for a baby, do a patch test first by gently rubbing a piece of dried or fresh chamomile on their skin before adding to a bath. Chamomile is a member of the ragweed family, so you want to see if there is an allergic reaction before bathing them in it. If there's no reaction, put chamomile into a small tea ball (about 1 tablespoon), boil 1 cup of water, and pour over the tea ball. Steep for about 6 minutes, then add the water to your baby's bathwater, making sure it isn't too hot. Make sure to pour over their head to cleanse them energetically.

For teething, soak a clean washcloth in diluted chamomile tea, pop in the fridge to cool, and give to your baby to suck on before bed or once during the day. This reduces inflammation and eases the pain.

....

Clarity Bath

This bath is helpful for clearing up your energy and casting out anything you've held on to from negative interactions. It is a simple mixture of cascarilla, honey, and holy water, although some opt for Florida water instead.

½ ounce cascarilla from a botanica, crushed with a mortar and pestle to turn it back into a powder

Drizzle of honey

Splash of holy water

Fill a basin with water and mix in the cascarilla. Add the honey and the holy water. As you mix everything with your hands, speak into the water. Tell it the purpose of this bath is for cleansing and clearing. When finished, pour this over your head and body. This can be done on a regular basis as needed.

....

Honey Rose Bath

This bath is for adults but can also be used for babies, as it is sweetening and filled with loving vibrations.

A white candle

Petals of 2 dozen fresh organic roses (pink for self-love, yellow for joy, or traditional red)

A few drops of honey

Splash of Florida water

Splash of rosewater

Optional: rose-infused oil

Light the candle before you begin. Either steep the rose petals in a ½ gallon of hot water or break up the rose petals and immerse them in cold water in a basin. Pray to bring in sweetness, a more loving connection with self, the protection of unconditional love, or loving vibrations in all your relationships. As you do this, add the honey, the Florida water, and the rosewater. Pour this mixture over your body while standing in the tub. Air-dry and moisturize with the rose-infused oil.

For a baby, light the candle, steep the rose petals in 4 cups of hot water, then add the honey, Florida water, and rosewater. Pray into it, infusing it with your intentions. Strain, and allow to cool to warm but not too hot. Using a sponge, soak up some of the mixture and gently pour it over the baby's body and head (avoiding the eyes and mouth). Afterward, either allow baby to air-dry or gently pat with a towel. Rub them down with the rose-infused oil afterward. Make sure to follow up with lots of snuggles and love-filled kisses.

Lavender, Rose, and Chamomile Bath

This bath is for babies, to calm, soothe, and cleanse them; cover them with sweet, loving energy; and protect them. Adults can use it during pregnancy and postpartum.

1 cup (for adults), or ½ tablespoon (for babies), dried lavendar

1 cup (for adults), or ½ tablespoon (for babies), dried rose

1 cup (for adults), or ½ tablespoon (for babies), dried chamomile

Splash of holy water

Sprinkle of cascarilla

Optional: a white candle

Place the lavender, rose, and chamomile in a small tea ball. Place the tea ball in a basin. Boil 1 cup of water and pour over; allow to steep for 6 minutes. Add the holy water and the cascarilla to the basin, then pour into baby's bathwater. You can light a white candle while doing this and praying/speaking your intentions into it. If using for adults, boil a ½ gallon of water and pour over the herbs. Steep for 6 minutes. Strain and allow to cool before pouring over yourself. This is one bath you could also add to the tub for yourself if you want the physical benefits to help ease your body.

....

Sweet Mint and Lavender Bath

This bath is for adults or bigger children. It sweetens the energy while being protective and uplifting. Additionally, it is soothing to the spirit and body.

1 bundle fresh peppermint (about 3 ounces)

Drizzle of honey

Splash of lavender cologne

Break up the fresh peppermint in a ½ gallon of cold water, or break up and steep in hot water for a few minutes if preparing for children. Add the honey and the lavender cologne; stir clockwise with your hand to call in sweetness and tenderness. Strain and allow to cool before pouring on your head or over your/their body.

....

Sunshine Bath

This bath is for vitality, strength, joy, and protection. It is suitable for babies, children, and adults.

1 medium bundle chamomile

1 medium bundle calendula

1 medium bouquet sunflowers, flowers cut from stems

Splash of holy water

A yellow or white candle

For babies, you can use enough chamomile and calendula from the bundle to fill a small tea ball. Then steep the tea ball in 4 cups of hot water. Place the flowers in the water. Add the holy water. Light the candle and pray for strength, joy, vitality, and protection. Use a sponge to pour the water over the baby's body while praying over them or speaking words of affirmation.

For adults, light the candle, then immerse the herbs and flowers in a basin of water, breaking up what you can and praying. Add the holy water, then strain the liquid. Pour over yourself while standing in the bathtub or shower. Additionally, you could add this to your bathwater in the tub if you wish to experience the physical benefits for itchy skin.

Note: This bath is for postpartum and is not to be used during pregnancy, as calendula can cause miscarriage.

....

Be The Peace Bath

This bath can be used for all ages to balance emotions and bring a sense of peace.

½ cup lavender

Splash of agua de violetas cologne

Sprinkle of cascarilla

A blue candle

Pour 8 ounces of boiling water over the lavender. Steep for 6 minutes. Strain into a basin and allow to cool. Add the agua de violetas cologne and the cascarilla. Work them in with your hands while focusing on peaceful thoughts. Light the candle and place it in the center of the basin. Pray over it, calling in peace and tranquility. Visualize a blue light filling the water, infusing it with even more calming energies. When it's cooled, either add this to your baby's bathwater or pour over your or your older child's head.

....

THE SOAKS

Citrus Soak

This soak is cleansing and energizing.

1 organic lemon

1 organic lime

1 organic grapefruit

1 bundle of basil
   (about 3 ounces)

1 cup Epsom salt

2 white candles

1 brown paper bag

Wash and slice the citrus fruits and rip up the basil. Fill your bathtub with warm water. Add the Epsom salt, slices of fruit, and basil into the bath. Light the candles and place them at either end of your tub. Set the brown paper bag outside of the tub within reach. Get in the bath and pray for cleansing and rejuvenation. Meditate on what has been stressing you and visualize it dissolving like the salt in the bath. Anything that has been weighing on you, release it. If your pregnancy has been tiring, visualize your body charging up and filling with strength. Take a slice of the fruit and rub your whole body with it, visualizing it absorbing any excess energy weighing you down. When finished, discard in the brown paper bag.

....

Cucumber Soak

This soak relieves itchy pregnancy skin and soothes and cools emotions.

1 cucumber, peeled and sliced   Optional: bath oil

Magnesium oil or spray

Add the cucumber slices to a lukewarm bath. Add a bath oil of your choosing (optional); just be cautious about getting slippery. Soak for at least thirty minutes, rubbing the cucumber slices on your body where you are itchy. When finished, pat dry or air-dry and follow up with magnesium oil or spray on your legs.

....

Oatmeal Soak

This soak soothes itchy skin and is baby-safe.

2 cups organic oats

2 cups (for adults), or 1 cup (for babies), goat milk or coconut milk

3 tablespoons (for adults), or 1 tablespoon (for babies), organic honey or skin-grade manuka honey

Pure shea butter

Blend oats in blender until they're a powder, then add to a lukewarm bath. Add the honey and the goat milk or coconut milk. Soak for 20 to 30 minutes. For a baby, soak for 10 to 15 minutes. Pat dry and moisturize with pure shea butter. If you are concerned about using honey with your baby, feel free to omit it, or wash their hands after and avoid getting the soak on their face.

....

Detox Soak

Detox baths are becoming more and more popular these days, for everything from relieving heavy metal buildup to cleansing negative energies. They can also be grounding and healing for your skin. If using with your baby, I suggest waiting until they are at least three months old to avoid irritating their sensitive newborn skin. If your child is older, you can add a splash of apple cider vinegar as well, but I wouldn't recommend it for an infant or toddler.

1 teaspoon Epsom salt   1 teaspoon baking soda
½ teaspoon bentonite clay

Add all ingredients to the bathwater in your baby's tub. Mix thoroughly using your hands. Place your baby in and allow them to soak in it for 15 minutes. You can rinse them off with clean water if you'd like, or you can pat dry and moisturize. I prefer to rinse with clean warm water and then moisturize so that anything that was released is not left on them.

Note: This soak should only be done postpartum or prior to conception.

....

OIL BLENDS

Make or purchase these oil blends to anoint yourself or your baby with extra loving goodness. They can also be used to alleviate certain skin conditions.

While following the preparations below, remember to infuse your oil with your intention. Once your blend is sealed in its jar, speak life into it, pray over it, and visualize your energy flowing into it to charge it up.

Liquid Sunshine Blend

This oil is calming, soothing, and offers strength in times of need. I have found it to be uplifting when I'm feeling down as well. The amounts of herbs and oil will vary based on the size of the jar you use.

A sterile glass jar
Dried calendula
Dried chamomile
Dried sunflower

Carrier oil of your choice
(sunflower, avocado, olive)
Vitamin E capsules

In the jar, place equal parts dried calendula, dried chamomile, and dried sunflower. Cover the herbs with the carrier oil—there should be at least 1 inch of oil above the dried herbs and 1 to 3 inches of room at the top of the jar.

This blend is best infused by the sun, so seal the jar and then either place it in a brown paper bag or wrap it in a cloth. Place it in a sunny spot and shake it up a few times a day. Do this for 1 to 2 weeks and then strain with a cheesecloth over a fine mesh strainer.

Pour into a sterile jar (or jars) and add the oil from a split vitamin E capsule as a preservative. Label the jar with the date. Infused oils can last up to 2 years, depending on your preparation and storage. I typically suggest checking on it after 1 month of use (because life happens and sometimes our storage isn't perfectly executed). You'll notice if it smells off or has gone rancid and should not continue to be used. I prefer not to add any essential oils or fragrance, but follow your intuition if you feel called to. This is safe for little ones and can be soothing for rashes and eczema. After infusing, keep out of direct sunlight.

Note: This oil blend should only be used prior to conception or during postpartum because of the calendula.

....

The Power of Love Blend

This oil is filled with loving energy and sweetness while offering protection. It is safe for use on little ones and throughout pregnancy. It is also a sensual oil that is perfect for massages. The amounts of ingredients will vary based on the size of the jar you use.

1 pod vanilla

Two sterile glass jars

Dried rose

Dried white geranium

Carrier oil of your choice
  (sunflower, avocado, olive)

1 vitamin E capsule

Slice the vanilla pod down the middle and remove the seeds, or chop the pod into chunks. Place seeds or chunks in one of the jars and add equal parts dried rose and dried white geranium. Cover the herbs with the carrier oil—there should be at least 1 inch of oil above the dried herbs and 1 to 3 inches of room at the top of the jar. Give it a good shake before filling a saucepan a quarter of the way with water. Place the ring of a mason jar lid on the bottom of the pan before putting the jar in. This helps prevent the glass from breaking. Simmer for 6 hours. When finished, strain with a cheesecloth through a mesh strainer. Label a separate sterile jar with the date, pour in the oil, and add the oil of the vitamin E capsule. This blend should be good for a year, but I always err on the side of caution and keep an eye on it after 1 month.

....

CHAPTER 10

NAVIGATING TRAUMA

I n such an emotionally open and vulnerable time as pregnancy and the postpartum period, trauma, even trauma that we think we've healed or moved on from, can make itself known again. We can also experience and carry trauma in our bodies from pregnancy, birth, and postpartum. Old wounds show up during conception, pregnancy, birth, and postpartum. Your trauma may not show for every single experience, but it will be an uninvited guest at times.

How we navigate this is deeply personal. You've probably heard to be gentle with yourself and extend yourself grace. But what does this look like? Sometimes it looks like not shaming ourselves if we're not excited about pregnancy the way someone else would be. Other times, it looks like accepting that our response to childbirth may not look like what's portrayed in happy movies. It can also look like allowing ourselves to fall apart instead of forcing ourselves to hold it together. We may try to control things to avoid being triggered instead of creating an approach based on the reality that our trauma may emerge anyway, and not because something went "wrong." Even the most seemingly straightforward pregnancy or birth can lead to sensations that remind us of a traumatic event. The pain we experience during labor and the inability to control it or just make it stop can trigger us. Some things are not in anyone's control, which is why being gentle with ourselves, instead of punishing ourselves for our response, is important.

Having the difficult but necessary conversations with our partner and birth team ahead of time is essential. We generally do not feel good talking about our trauma or even know how to begin. It brings up so many feelings that we think we have buried deep enough that we won't experience unexpected reminders. We may anticipate not receiving the response we need or hope for because that is what happened in the past. It is important to do it anyway, so that you can create a plan that properly supports you.

When I was pregnant, I did not fully disclose my trauma related to sexual assault and create a plan around it with my birth team. The cervical exam during labor was triggering, and I experienced it multiple times over the course of a few days. The second time, we had to stop partway through and begin again because I could not breathe. This was my body's response to the memory of the trauma that resides in me. Fortunately, my partner, mom, midwife, doula, and I were able to communicate in the moment and figure out how to proceed in a way that was doable for me. They were all grounding and supportive and recognized what was going on. Still, I wish I had been more honest with myself about the fact that my trauma might come up during labor. I have a high tolerance for pain and was so focused on affirming to myself and my body that I would be "good at birth" and avoiding a negative inner dialogue that I forgot to honor my body's truth—that trauma still lives here.

A high tolerance for pain and a mind-over-matter approach is only going to do so much when your body responds to the memory of trauma it has tucked away. Your birth team can remind you in those moments that you are safe and have autonomy over your body, and help you to pace things in a way that you can process safely.

No matter how informed we may be or how well versed in our mind's or body's response to our past experiences, things change. We can unearth new triggers, new responses. As we evolve, as our life changes, so does the way we experience the trauma that resides in our minds and bodies. Healing work doesn't remove the trauma, but it can shift how we are able to respond when it presents itself. Think of the way that therapy focuses on presenting new thought pathways for us to take; it doesn't remove the thought pathways that aren't helpful. Instead, it gives us new ones that we can choose to go down. It's up to us to take the steps. We won't get it right every time, but we can do our best to try.

Finding a trauma-informed doctor, therapist, or healer can feel daunting. Many of us think the people who occupy these roles should already be equipped with the ability to guide us. Unfortunately, this isn't the case. The simplest way is to inquire about their understanding of all the ways trauma impacts our lives and experiences. Do they understand the physical effects or only the mental? Do they understand how it changes the way you experience certain things—in this case, pregnancy and childbirth? Treat it like an interview, and don't be shy about asking questions.

If you have had trauma in your past that you think might reemerge in the pregnancy or childbirth process, some ways to navigate it are:

- Finding creative outlets as a way to release and express what you can't say. This can be done in a way that feels safer and more doable than speaking your experience out loud; think drawing, writing, painting, or beadwork.

- Learning different ways to soothe and calm your central nervous system, such as EFT tapping; breathwork exercises/practices; meditation; and grounding methods, such as the "5-4-3-2-1" technique: identifying five things you can see, four things you can touch, three things you can hear, two things you can smell, and one thing you can taste, which brings you back to center and the present moment.

- Creating plans with your care teams about what to do in the event you're triggered—it's not just about prevention.

- Giving yourself grace and working on releasing your expectations of what a "good" pregnancy or birth looks like.

- Journaling to get things off your chest and out of your head.

- Connecting with a counselor, therapist, or healer.

- Getting active to help move any stagnant energy in your body with dance, yoga, jogging, walking, or whatever feels good to you.

- Reminding yourself that while trauma can at times leave us feeling consumed by it, you are more than your trauma.

- Being honest about ways in which systemic oppression played a role in your traumatic experience, and releasing any guilt you have internalized.

- Taking things moment by moment instead of day by day.

AFFIRMATIONS

- I am more than my past experiences.

- The goal of healing is not to be a person unaffected by trauma but to be able to cope productively.

- My trauma is a part of my life experiences, but it is not who I am.

CHAPTER 11

INTUITION
VS. ANXIETY

While I was pregnant, my anxiety mostly went out the window. It popped up occasionally, but otherwise, for the first time in a long time, I wasn't anxious. I was completely consumed by my pregnancy, in a place of bliss and excitement. My intuition was even more potent and crystal clear. This isn't the case for everyone. While your intuition may be heightened, you may also be anxious, and understandably so. This can muddy the waters when you're trying to decipher the messages you're receiving. Learning to differentiate between the two—intuition and anxiety—can feel confusing. Everyone says to listen to your gut, but maybe anxiety has taken your gut by the reins and ridden off into the sunset. So how do you tune in to that intuition that becomes enhanced in pregnancy and comes with parenthood? Before you try to quiet your mind, learn which narrative/ voice is which. There's no sense in fighting to quiet the mind if then you're unsure of the source for what's coming through.

Anxiety can be all-consuming in the way it can create so many worst-case scenarios and a sense of impending doom (which it then spends every moment trying to convince you is inevitable and in fact already happening). Anxiety comes from a place of fear and works overtime. Learning to identify this voice/narrative is important because when you recognize that it's anxiety doing all the talking, you can respond accordingly. Take note of how repetitive the thoughts are and how much of a web is being spun to get you stuck, not just mentally but even physically, because anyone who's experienced serious anxiety knows how debilitating it can be. Anxiety spends a moment coming up with the worst of the worst, and every other waking (and sleeping, if you can get any) moment convincing you it will happen. Learn to recognize this voice, and know that while it's well-intentioned—it's your mind's way of trying to protect you from the harm it perceives—it is misguided. If you've spent much of your life waiting for the other shoe to drop, this may feel like you're going against all you know. Remember this: seasons change, and what we need and what works for us in one season likely won't in the next. Wearing a bubble coat in the winter is helpful, but wearing one in the summer because you're waiting for a snowy day is not.

Intuition is less demanding than anxiety, but not every message is one of sunshine and rainbows. Intuition is straightforward, simple, and clear. It may tell you something isn't safe or bring a warning, but it will not bring fear into you. Intuition is confident and solid. You'll be able to take direct action instead of feeling consumed with fear of what is to come. We've all had moments where we felt a pull or heard a voice telling us not to go to an event, only to find out the next day that we avoided some drama or issue by staying home. The way this differs from anxiety is the dialogue. Intuition simply says, "Nope," while anxiety spins you into a web of a million reasons, most of which aren't even plausible. Learn to hear the clear, strong, and direct voice of intuition. Honor it when you do, and it will become stronger each time.

For some people, their gut hasn't always been a reliable compass. Trauma can lead the body to signal that everything is a threat, even things that aren't. Or sometimes the body signals that everything is okay when it isn't, simply because it is familiar. When trying to home in on your intuition, once again ask yourself:

Where is this response coming from? Is it coming from a place of familiarity? Is it coming from a place of fear? Is it coming from a place outside of your body? When I had trouble differentiating due to my own trauma, it helped me the most to make note of whether it was my body signaling me or something beyond it. When it was beyond my body and I took action accordingly, I wasn't misled.

One way to work with your intuition during pregnancy (or anytime) is by using oracle or tarot cards. This can help you to make better sense of things if you're having a hard time. Prayer is powerful, too. Take it to your altar; consult your ancestors and spirit guides. Ask for them to bring you clarity in a dream or to give you a sign. Unfortunately, many herbs for psychic enhancement and intuition support are not safe for pregnancy. Try working with them in the form of a scented candle or incense instead, and meditating or working with oracle/tarot cards. You can also use dried versions of the herbs in a sachet placed either in your pillowcase or on your person/in your pocket.

Consider anointing your third eye with lavender oil to support your intuition while offering protection. You can also try wearing purple, which is associated with but not limited to intuition, psychic abilities, and divination. There are many ways to work with your enhanced intuition that are simple, practical, and pregnancy-safe.

Don't write off keeping a dream journal, especially considering some pregnancy dreams are bizarre. Keeping a journal can help make sense of your dreams and, combined with intentional dream work, help you to use them as visions. Try this bedtime exercise, plus a sachet of mugwort, lavender, and jasmine in your pillowcase, to promote visions in your dreams.

Bedtime ritual: Before you hop into bed, get your space prepared. Avoid clutter and chaos, such as laundry dumped everywhere, knickknacks out of place, etc. Burn jasmine incense. Get in a comfortable position on your bed and begin with grounding. Visualize yourself as a tree, with your body as the trunk and roots extending from you into the ground, connecting you and grounding you to the physical realm and the magnetic energy of the earth. When you feel good and ready, call on your spiritual team. Begin to count down from ten with the intention of visualizing them when you reach one. Slowly allow them to come into your mind's eye. Greet them, and discuss with them what it is you'd like to dream about or receive clarity about through your dreams tonight. Ask that they reveal to you all that you need to know and that they place a shield of protection around you as you sleep. Thank them, and when you're ready, open your eyes. Snuff out the jasmine incense and go to sleep. When you wake up in the morning, record any dreams in your dream journal. While they may not make sense, give it a grace period—time has a way of revealing all. You may also experience immediate clarity, so be prepared for this. While we may ask for clarity about something, it doesn't always mean we're as ready as we think for the big reveal.

Years before I was pregnant, my guides repeatedly tried to get a message to me about someone I was involved with. I foolishly dismissed it because, well, it wasn't what I wanted to believe to be true. Eventually, though, I asked that they reveal to me the evidence connected to what they were saying. In a dream, they not only revealed it but warned me that since I had not listened earlier, I wouldn't need to look any further because it would be arriving on my doorstep. It did, and it brought with it a drama-filled day. There's a common scene you've probably seen played out in movies and in life where a woman has a dream her partner is cheating (and they are), and she spends the day mad at them instead of honoring the vision and leaving. We have to be careful what we ask for, because, while fortunately, I was ready to do what I had to do, sometimes we're not.

HERBAL SUGGESTIONS

- **Jasmine:** Try as either a candle or the dried herb in a sachet in your pillowcase for dream work.

- **Yarrow:** Use dried in a sachet, either in your pillowcase or in your pocket, for psychic dreams and enhanced psychic abilities.

- **Mugwort:** Use dried in a sachet, for protection and psychic enhancement placed in your pillowcase.

- **Lavender:** Use dried in a sachet and hung above your bed or placed in your pillowcase, for psychic protection and support. Can also be burned as a bundle or as incense.

AFFIRMATIONS

- My intuition is a natural part of me that I connect with wholeheartedly.

- I release what no longer serves me well from previous seasons of my life.

- My mind may be foggy at times, and my heart may put rose-tinted glasses on my eyes, but my intuition does not lie.

MEDITATIONS

These meditations are ones I crafted and used in my pregnancy. I have shared them with clients to support them in their pregnancies as well. My personal tip is to record yourself (in your voice notes app or with a camera) reciting them. Then play the meditation of your choosing so you can follow along. This makes for a much more seamless experience than constantly opening your eyes to read the next part in the book. Eventually you will be able to do them without the recording.

MEDITATION FOR CONNECTING WITH YOUR BABY

Center yourself and light a candle to represent the bond between you two. (If you are having multiples, do this separately for each baby. You can do this over several days or times of day to accommodate.) Take three deep breaths—as deep as your reduced lung capacity will allow—unclench your jaw, drop your shoulders, soften your hips, and allow your body to relax.

Close your eyes and visualize yourself in a brightly lit hallway. At the end of the hallway is a door; on the other side of the door is a room where your baby is. Begin counting down from ten as you walk down the hall, opening the door when you get to one. As you step into the room, you and your baby are the only ones there. The energy is warm and inviting; there's a rocking chair next to a bassinet where your baby is lying down. Approach the bassinet and connect with your baby's energy before picking them up. When ready, pick them up and sit in the rocking chair with them. Share with your baby the birthing plan and ask if there is anything they need from you. Ask if there is anything they feel fearful of. Make note of their response; there is no right or wrong.

If you are hoping for your baby to move into a better position for labor, as you rock in the chair, let the baby know what you'll be doing to help them change their position, and ask that they work with you. Help them to understand it is for the best, and that they'd be surprised just how comfortable it is to be in that position. Be encouraging, and share how much you love them already.

When you are ready, let them know that soon enough they'll be in your arms, and though it will be different from being in the womb, just like in the womb, you'll be together. Place the baby back in the bassinet and begin to walk back to the door. When you open the door, count up to ten, walking through the hallway and back to your present space. When you feel you are done, open your eyes and say, "This meditation is now complete and closed." Then snuff out the candle. This is done to close the connection, similar to hanging up the phone. You can always call back.

MEDITATION AND RITUAL FOR PROTECTION

Light a small white or black candle dressed with dried rosemary, dried basil, and crushed bay leaves. To dress the candle, anoint it with olive oil or protection oil purchased from a botanica. Then roll it in the dried herbs. Take a moment to center yourself. Take three deep breaths in, and release more tension from your body with each breath out. With eyes closed, visualize a bright bubble of blue light in your center. Watch as it begins to grow, slowly but surely, until you are surrounded by the bubble. Feel the warmth, the protection, the strength of it. Be present for the moment. Nothing can harm you. When you feel ready, visualize branches of a rosebush, its many thorns going outward. These branches make a shield around the bubble, arching over it and you. Repeat the following out loud: "Through the power of my highest spirit guides and all that is divine, I am protected in all ways, at all times." Continue to focus on the branches and the bubble. Feel them getting stronger as you do. When you feel all is complete, come back to the present moment and open your eyes. Thank your spirits, ancestors, and creator for their assistance in this. Let the candle burn down completely.

You can do this for your baby as well. Simply visualize the bubble and branches covering your baby instead. Change "I" to your baby's name in the incantation. You can do this with your baby present or even before they're born. Eventually teach your children to do this meditation (always supervise any lit candle).

MEDITATION FOR SLEEP

This meditation is the best for helping you to gain better control of the mind-body connection. It is one my dad taught me as a child, and while it may not be the most exciting, it is simple and effective.

While lying in bed, close your eyes and take three deep breaths. Release any tension in your body as best you can. In your mind's eye, visualize yourself in a classroom with a chalkboard. Walk up to the chalk-board and write with a piece of chalk the number one hundred. Visualize yourself erasing the number, then write ninety-nine. Erase once again. Repeat this until you have gotten to zero or fallen asleep. Should you make it to zero, start over from one hundred again.

With time, you won't make it past ninety, or even ten, which, during pregnancy, can be a godsend considering how difficult it is to get to sleep some nights. This is also a meditation you can eventually share with your children, as part of wind-down time before bed.

TREE MEDITATION

When connecting with a tree for grounding, or to take a load off emotionally, always bring an offering, such as bread, fruit, or coins. Visualize your energy and the tree's energy connecting with each other, circulating between you two, flowing together and communicating with one another. Feel the tree grounding you and tell the tree your problems. Do this while you have at least one hand on the tree. Try hugging it. Feel yourself becoming soothed, the weight coming off your chest as you share. Allow the tree to share with you any wisdom as it takes the load off. Always give thanks.

If you're doing this for grounding, visualize roots coming out of your feet and connecting to the root system of the tree. Feel the strength of the roots keeping you both grounded. You're able to sway with the wind, weather the storm, and still remain in place. Do this until you feel it's complete. Thank the tree.

SHOWER MEDITATION

This simple meditation releases tension, stress, and excess energies. In the shower, begin by relaxing and counting down from twenty. Take deep breaths and release as the water pours onto your head. Soften your brow, unclench your jaw, drop your shoulders, and soften your stomach and pelvic area. Relax your hips, soften your leg muscles, and feel all the tension leaving your body through your feet. Focus on the warmth of the water soothing you, washing energy down, and easing your aching muscles. Visualize yourself being energized through the crown of your head, throughout your body. Push out any residual energy that isn't serving your highest good.

When you're ready to wash your body, work from the neck down to take away any energy you need to release or remove. After, say, "I release all energy that does not serve my highest good," and rinse. Traditionally you would then lather up again from the bottom up, but this can be difficult when pregnant. If you're able to, call in sweet and strong energy as you do this.

If you aren't, that's okay, too; honor your body. Before stepping out of the shower, say out loud three times, "My energetic field is now sealed." Dress in light-colored clothing for the rest of the day.

ELEPHANT VISUALIZATION

Get into a comfortable position and take a moment to center yourself. Take three deep breaths, bringing each breath deeper into your core. Continue to take deep breaths at a rate comfortable for you. Close your eyes and count down from twenty. With each number, use your mind's eye to visualize open plains. Twenty, nineteen, eighteen, seventeen—feel the ground beneath your feet—sixteen, fifteen, fourteen—the sun shining down on you—thirteen, twelve, eleven—the breeze blowing across your face—ten, nine, eight—the smell of the grass—seven, six, five—see an elephant standing in front of you—four, three, two—it's just you and the elephant—and one. You and the elephant are standing on the plains. You are both calm. Take a moment to connect with her and her spirit. Feel her strength, her grace, her wisdom, and take it all in.

When ready, slowly approach her, focusing on your breath as you do. Watch as your breathing and hers come in sync. Raise your hand up as she brings her head down for you. Gently place your hand on her forehead; feel her warmth. Ask her to share with you her wisdom for birth, and for your birthing experience specifically. Let the first thing that comes to mind just flow in; that is your answer. There is no right or wrong, just embrace the wisdom she has to share. Ask any questions you may have. Be open to receiving, even if it's difficult to hear. Ask for her to give you strength and support when it comes time for birth. Ask that she and her herd surround you and protect you from harm. That they sound the trumpets if something goes wrong. Give her thanks and love. Ask where and how to leave an offering for her, if she wants one at all.

When done, count up from one and go your separate ways. One, two, three—you begin to come back to your present surroundings—four, five, six—the plains begin to fade—seven, eight, nine—she begins to fade as well—ten, eleven, twelve—you are coming back to the present—thirteen, fourteen, fifteen—she's off in the distance—sixteen, seventeen, eighteen—the plains have faded completely—nineteen, twenty. Open your eyes. Take your time before getting up; write down any messages from the elephant. If she gave you instructions for how to leave an offering, do what you can to prepare that for her.

BIRTH/LABOR
MEDITATION #1

This meditation is to be used during labor, and during birth if possible. Call on your honorable guides and ancestors to ask that they come forth to assist you. Call on them for strength and for protection as this new soul is being brought earth-side. Close your eyes; visualize them holding your baby (or babies) and ushering them down the birth canal and into the world. Breathe with your contractions and breathe down into your pelvis. Allow this breath to push the baby along. When faced with resistance, do not bear down—continue to take deep breaths. Visualize your honorable guides and ancestors supporting you in whatever position you're in. Feel their strength supporting you, feel their energy helping you to ride each contraction. Breathe into your body and allow your muscles to loosen with each breath and release. Ask them to assist you with grounding your energy. Thank them as they help ease you through each contraction. Do this for as long as you can or is necessary. This meditation is kept simple so as to keep you focused on the task at hand rather than feeling overwhelmed in the moment.

BIRTH/LABOR
MEDITATION #2

Focus on your breathing and visualize yourself as a tree. The many roots that come out underneath you are your honorable guides and ancestors. They are keeping you connected and centered and giving you strength. They communicate with you through these roots. Feel them, embrace them, use them to call on your guides and ancestors to lead you through this. As you continue to breathe, focus your vision on feeling solid even as a breeze is blowing. This breeze is each contraction you feel; it blows through your branches and may even cause you to sway. It does not uproot you, though. It passes, and you are still here. Focus in on your root system, and ask for your guides and ancestors to share any words of encouragement, wisdom, or guidance for the task at hand. If there are none, simply ask them to continue to give you strength and support, to continue to hold you down and guide you through this, even just energetically. Feel their strength flowing through you. Allow your branches and trunk to sway with the contractions, but remember your strength. Stay in this place until you need to come out; thank your guides and ancestors when you do.

CLEANSING AND
VISUALIZATION COMBO

Take a spiritual cologne of your choice or holy water. Pour some into your hands, rub them together, and run your hands in a sweeping motion over your head and body. Make sure to get the back of your neck, lower back, and feet. These are all entry points for energy and can also be where energy gets backed up. As you do this, visualize any negative energy leaving your auric field and body. Cast it out by saying out loud, "I release any energy that is not serving my highest good."

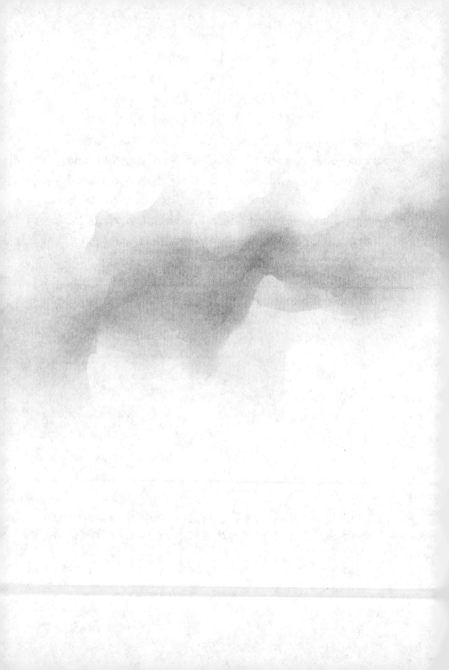

CHAPTER 13

YOUR AURA

We all have an aura, an energetic field that surrounds us. It can be filled with energy that we're emitting, and it can also take on energetic debris from interactions with others or psychic or energetic attacks. This is why it's important to cleanse and shield ourselves regularly. A simple way of doing this is by visualizing yourself in an impenetrable bubble. You can make the bubble a certain color, such as blue, pink, purple, green, indigo, ultraviolet, etc.—something that feels powerful and safe to you. While there are many other ways, this is a good starting point for those who are unfamiliar with the practice and need something straightforward and practical for daily use.

There can be holes in our aura from which people drain our energy. When you're feeling particularly depleted, seek out an energy worker you trust so they can seal it for you.

If you're curious to know more about yours, you can go for a reading. There are different types of aura readings, including aura photography. Your aura can change day to day, even moment to moment, but it's possible for it to be consistent. I know a few people whose aura always photographs as red, which reflects their passionate and powerful personalities. I know some whose aura always photographs as yellow and orange because of their creative and joyful attributes. What's beautiful about aura photography is that the picture can help you see what is going on energetically. Seeing auras without a camera is a skill that can be developed or strengthened over time, too, but if that's not your forte, it's beneficial to have it captured in a photo, as well as to be able to track how it has or hasn't changed over time. You can trace how you have grown energetically or stayed true to yourself despite what has been thrown at you.

During pregnancy, our aura reveals so much. It gives us insight into things we sometimes can't put words to. We can see how the pregnancy is impacting us energetically, beyond what we are feeling physically. Aura photos can also be a form of divination. I have seen pregnancies show up in aura photos, including mine, and even in a couple's aura photo. Energy is everything, though, so it's no surprise.

Pregnancy is such a spiritual experience, in ways

that the untrained eye cannot see. Being a witness to all the ways we develop over those nine months is a privilege. I frequently get my aura photographed, and when I was pregnant, I kept going over the trimesters. Just like my body was changing, my aura was, too, all in preparation for this baby and my own evolution. In the beginning, the physical toll was evident, but so was the grounded and protective stance I had taken. There was a lot of red and pink in my heart space. As time went on, my heart space, which always was lit up, was even more activated—brighter—showing the bonding happening with my baby. The crown of my head showed an even deeper spiritual connection and my enhanced psychic abilities (mother's intuition). As I shifted into the second trimester, my aura became blue, purple, pink, and green. In my third trimester, my throat was lit up, in preparation to advocate for my-self during birth and for my baby after. Everything I was experiencing emotionally and mentally could be seen clear as day in my energetic field.

If you happen to get your aura photographed while trying to conceive, look to where green shows up, if at all. Green is associated with abundance and fertility. Look for an orb of light, particularly if you're taking a couple's photo. This can be the baby's spirit showing up early to the party. Make note of what colors show up in your pelvic area. This will give you insight into what energy you're holding there or working with.

While there are slight variations in the color correspondences, especially in regard to where they are in the photo, what other colors accompany them, and if they are murky or dark, typically they are as follows:

- **Red:** Passion, power, strength, personal drive, grounded, anger, frustration, overworked, low energy

- **Orange:** Creative, positive, friendly, motivated

- **Yellow:** Joyful, confident, charismatic, optimistic, courageous

- **Green:** Healing, love, growth, change, opportunity

- **Blue:** Self-expression, inner balance, trust, peace

- **Purple:** Intuition, spiritual

- **Indigo:** Intuition, empathy, sensitive, healing abilities

- **Pink:** Love, kindness, nurturing, compassion

- **White:** Openness, oneness/sense of being whole, open-minded, possibility of overthinking, protection

- **Rainbow:** Depending on how it shows up, encompasses a balance of all the colors

The interpretation of how these show up in your photo and aura varies greatly because each aura is a personal and individual energetic field. No two will be exactly the same. The colors' placement also influences what they represent. The above is a loose guide to give you a base of understanding. Keep in mind, you may have other colors, such as magenta, that can occur when some of the colors blend together. What that means for you will be revealed in a reading.

Pay attention to what color is showing up around your throat in particular. This can indicate that you might have a difficult time with speaking up or advocating for yourself; if you know this is going to be a roadblock for you, you can begin working on it now, for you and your baby. What shows up in your crown area can reveal how your intuition is developing as time goes on. Often, we will find the affirmation of the work we've done, or the aura will reveal the work we may still need to do—such as your heart space becoming brighter or filled with green, indicating growth and love as it opens up during pregnancy. Orange may show up more as you create new life. It may also reveal just how taxing pregnancy can be in a murky red. Be open to the possibilities. Remember, it's a tool and you decide how you use it.

A beginner's way of seeing your aura, or others', is by first making sure there is soft lighting to avoid any energetic interference, extending your hand out in front of a white wall (or having the person you're observing sit/stand in front of a wall), focusing on a central point on your subject, then letting your eyes lose focus. You'll begin to see a glow around the person or your hand/arm. Allow the colors to be revealed to you. It may not happen immediately, and it takes time and practice, but keep trying. You can also do this with your peripheral vision by having your hand/arm or the person in your peripheral field as you soften your gaze.

Practitioners of energetic healing such as Reiki, pranic healing, and other forms are trained in ways to see and feel the aura. If you are a practitioner, feel free to do an auric check-in on yourself more regularly. Often we do this for clients but are not as diligent with ourselves. I highly recommend Magic Jewelry in NYC, as well as Radiant Human.

AFFIRMATIONS

- I am ever changing like my aura; of this, I am accepting.

- My aura reveals I am more than meets the eye.

- My energy clearly speaks for me.

CHAPTER 14

ASTROLOGY

Before I became pregnant the second time, not only did I feel it and see countless signs, but it came up in a birth chart reading. I wanted insight about my Saturn return—when Saturn comes back into the sign it was in when you were born, twenty-seven to thirty years later. It's known to be a time during which trustworthy guidance is paramount, because the way it affects your life is big. Some people have great difficulty during these years, and for some, it's a time they look back on fondly. As the astrologist was going through my chart, I could hear her tone change. She was excited but treading lightly because what she was about to reveal might not have been welcome news. She shared that I would be getting pregnant that summer. She also shared that the placements in my chart indicated the baby who was coming and I had been connected in a past life. I took immense comfort in knowing that my pregnancy was written in the stars, and so was our connection from many lifetimes ago.

You may already know that you're a Virgo or your partner is a Gemini, but astrology goes well beyond the sun sign. Your moon, rising, Venus, Mars, etc. signs all give you more information than just the horoscope you see in the Sunday paper. For example, your Venus can give insight into the way you love, the way your heart operates, and your empathy toward others. Your moon can lend understanding to your emotions that live beneath the surface. As parents, we want to be able to support our children as best we can. Sometimes a personalized guide to understanding them and the possible life events they'll experience can make all the difference. The way I see it, the more tools you have to connect with your child and understand them, the better. See what the stars and planets have to say. You can decide what you do with that information, if anything at all.

Below is a brief summary of what the planetary placements, houses, and zodiac signs represent in your chart.

SIGNS AND ELEMENTS

Each zodiac sign is essentially a constellation of stars represented by the signs.

- **CAPRICORN**: Goat/earth,
  born on or between 12/22 and 1/19

- **AQUARIUS**: Water bearer/air,
  born on or between 1/20 and 2/18

- **PISCES**: Fish/water,
  born on or between 2/19 and 3/20

- **ARIES**: Ram/fire,
  born on or between 3/21 and 4/19

- **TAURUS**: Bull/earth,
  born on or between 4/20 and 5/20

- **GEMINI**: Twins/air,
  born on or between 5/21 and 6/21

- **CANCER**: Crab/water,
  born on or between 6/22 and 7/22

- **LEO**: Lion/fire,
  born on or between 7/23 and 8/22

- **VIRGO**: Virgin/earth,
  born on or between 8/23 and 9/22

- **LIBRA**: Scales/air,
  born on or between 9/23 and 10/23

- **SCORPIO**: Scorpion/water,
  born on or between 10/24 and 11/21

- **SAGITTARIUS**: Archer centaur/fire,
  born on or between 11/22 and 12/21

HOUSES

Houses are different areas of life that hold their own energy.

- **FIRST HOUSE**: Self/identity, body/physical image

- **SECOND HOUSE**: Income, money, values, possessions, resources, skills

- **THIRD HOUSE**: Communication, siblings and extended family, day-to-day, peers/neighbors

- **FOURTH HOUSE**: Home life, foundation, parents, family

- **FIFTH HOUSE**: Children, creativity, romance, self-expression

- **SIXTH HOUSE**: Health, routines/work, wellness

- **SEVENTH HOUSE:** Contracts and commitments (marriage, partnerships, close connections, etc.)

- **EIGHTH HOUSE:** Intimacy, transformation, inheritances/other people's money

- **NINTH HOUSE:** Philosophy, education, travel, belief systems, adventure

- **TENTH HOUSE:** Social status, career, reputation, legacy, what you are known for to the public

- **ELEVENTH HOUSE:** Humanitarianism/activism, tech, friends, community, long-term goals

- **TWELFTH HOUSE:** Subconscious, secrets, intuition, spirituality, loss, mental health

PLACEMENTS

Planetary placements influence the energy that your houses have. They will be in a certain zodiac sign as they move through the constellations (as seen from Earth), which is why you will have a certain planet in a certain sign.

- **SUN:** Ego/self

- **MOON:** Emotions, maternal influence/figure

- **MERCURY:** Communication, awareness

- **VENUS:** Love, money, desires

- **MARS:** Conflict style, personal way of taking action/making things happen, passion

- **JUPITER:** Worldly views, education, expansion/ exploration, luck

- **SATURN:** Karma, authority, paternal/father–figure influences

- **URANUS:** Unique events, rebellion, originality

- **NEPTUNE:** Spirituality, dreams, inspiration, illusion, fears, goals

- **PLUTO:** Transformation, personal power, rebirth

- **RISING/ASCENDANT:** First impressions, "the mask we wear." While this is not a planet, it is considered a point and is an important part of our birth chart. It is commonly used in what is called your "big 3." The other two that make up your "big 3" are your sun and moon.

Note: What these reflect in your chart will vary depending on the combinations. Each astrologer also has their personal approach, so this is just meant to be a supportive foundation that is open to interpretation. Let your astrologer's personal touch be just that.

Astrology can give you insight not only into what's to come, but into yourself and your relationships in the here and now. Think of it as a road map; it won't let you know where the potholes are, but it can give you a strong foundation of understanding to start your journey. This can be exceptionally helpful for new parents. It's easy to feel overwhelmed with getting to know a new baby and trying to understand them as they grow. Astrology can be supportive when it comes to navigating the ups and downs. Having my baby's birth chart done was affirming for me, because so much of what I already knew was confirmed, from the past-life connection, to personality traits, to things I needed to be on top of and supportive of.

I always warn my clients that astrology doesn't allow us to bypass doing the work because "that's just the way it is." Sure, having certain placements can explain why someone communicates the way they do or why they are more likely to be stubborn, but it doesn't mean these aren't things to work on or develop over time. I knew that, as a Sagittarius sun, I would be well equipped to support my child who has an Aries sun. We share the element of fire, so I can relate to so much that will impact my child as they grow up, such as their sense of self and how they'll express themselves. Fire signs are too often labeled as having bad tempers and being feisty, extra, loud, and so on. What's under that fiery exterior, though, is misunderstood passion and big hearts that lead us to be protective and vocal in ways others aren't. How this is seen by others is where things get complicated. I grew up in a house where I was the only fire sign. My father's sun was in an earth sign, and my mother and brother both had their suns in air signs. It was difficult to feel seen without having to constantly explain myself. While this led to my being good at communicating who I am and articulating how I wanted to be seen, it took a toll. Knowing that my child won't have to do that is something I'm happy about. We both also have air rising signs, which represent how the world sees you. We're curious, talkative, and on to the next thing as the wind changes. In a child, this can be interpreted by some adults as being nosy or the type who's always getting into trouble, needy, etc. Knowing how to support your kid beyond how they view themselves and through the lens of how the world sees them, and understanding their deeper, underlying emotions, is really a game changer, particularly when you can do that from birth.

If you're having difficulty figuring out your baby, a birth chart reading can be helpful in understanding what they came into this world with. Down the line, when you have a teenager whom you desperately want to connect with, their birth chart can help with that, too. You'll be able to better understand what they're working through emotionally, how they love or crush, how they handle conflict, and what karmic lessons they may be healing from in this lifetime. Now, as I said, a birth chart is simply a road map, and sometimes there are detours and potholes that you can't see ahead of time. It can guide you in many ways, but it can only do so much. Whatever your or your baby's chart says, trust your intuition above all when figuring out the best way to engage.

AFFIRMATIONS

- The stars don't lie, but even when they are read by the best guides, there is more than meets the eye.

- My baby's chart helps to prepare me to be their greatest ally.

- I will not limit my baby to what their star sign describes.

CHAPTER 15

PAST LIVES

The concept of past lives is not exclusive to one particular culture or belief. Each lifetime is an opportunity to grow and elevate our spirit. We choose the layout of our destiny before we agree to come back, creating and signing spiritual contracts. Now, of course, there will always be some things that are unaccounted for, such as the lessons of others' lifetimes that may intersect with ours. Since we are spiritual beings having a human experience, we need to go through the human side of things, which includes the unknown. That being said, we can always make decisions in this life that take us off the path we chose for ourselves, or create one that is more aligned with how we've elevated on a soul level in our current lifetime. That is part of free will. We also have the free will to step back onto our original path.

Years ago, a client of mine wanted to do some past-life healing, so we set up a regression session. During this session, we accessed memories from a lifetime before this one. She learned she had been a priestess who had a relationship with a member of a royal family: the queen. Not only as her personal high priestess, but a romantic one. Much of their time together was spent in secrecy, and while in some ways she accepted it, she wanted to be more than something kept in the shadows. Eventually, she made peace with their situation. In this lifetime, she still hid her talents, being low-key and reserved. She showed one persona on the outside and had another, private one inside. It held her back from taking chances on herself and going for what she truly wanted.

After our healing session, she shared how so much had been confirmed for her, down to why she didn't think she should publicly share her gifts. Not long after, she told me that she was finally going to put herself out there. No more hiding. This transformed her life completely. Had she been given this support long before, she would have already been sharing her light with the world. (That said, it's never too late to start, and one can say she simply followed the timeline that was in her path in the here and now.)

I have another client and colleague whom I've done

many past-life regressions with over the years. One in particular was connected to a pregnancy that she had terminated in this lifetime. She was filled with so much guilt and said she knew there was a past-life connection. We decided to investigate. During the regression, it was revealed that she had been a father to this baby's spirit in a past life. The child was born out of wedlock, and while in that lifetime, she promised the mother she would take care of the child, she did not. Instead, she sent the child off, to protect the "integrity" of her family line. The child died not long after. There was no guilt, shame, or feeling bad about not honoring the promise in that lifetime. But an energetic contract had been made all the same, one that the woman and the child had held her to. During this regression session, we facilitated healing for everyone involved and negotiated a new contract. While it may have seemed on the surface that the way to take care of that baby in this lifetime would be to give birth (because she is now more caring, more mindful), that wasn't the case. The baby would not have been better off being born at this moment in her life. The way that she could take care of her this time was by not bringing her into this world. This was for a number of reasons, from her health to her life circumstance and her emotional preparedness. She was tasked, though, with not forgetting her and making an effort to honor the baby's spirit by praying for its elevation. You may wonder why the baby's spirit came to her again if it wasn't the right time to come into this physical realm. It's because in this lifetime she has done the work that made it so she would care and right previous wrongs. Funnily enough, she had been told many times during spiritual ceremonies and masses that there was a little girl with her. Each time, she was adamant she had no idea who this little girl was. It was now clear that this baby's spirit had been with her since she came into this world (which makes sense even on a scientific level, considering we are born with all our eggs). This was an opportunity for them to heal, and they did. Sometimes, that is the reason a baby comes into our lives, to heal a past-life connection, and the how is different for every one of us. This past life took place over a thousand years ago. All this time had gone by, and still, they were connected.

Content warning: sexual assault.

One of my own past lives—one that has ongoing resonance in my life today—was traumatic. I had a husband and a child who were killed by invaders. I was assaulted, which led to another pregnancy. This child was taken from me by the descendants of those very same invaders. I spent the rest of that life searching for her. I live through the impact of these events every day, from my distrust of others to some of my desire to be a mother. I never forgave myself for what had happened, even though it was out of my hands. (I still get fixated on the coulda, woulda, shoulda.) The healing work my elder guided me through ultimately helped me to step into motherhood with strength. It helped me to feel worthy of being my child's mother once again. In many ways, I know this is one of the reasons why we were reunited. That we're getting another chance, because I finally forgave myself for what my child had already forgiven me for so many lifetimes ago. This shows how sometimes spiritual contracts we've made can be connected to our journey to parenthood—including what could possibly be preventing it on a spiritual level.

My views on what happens when our soul makes decisions before coming into this world are not the same as what many teach regarding past lives. They are my own. I don't believe that we choose our lives with the intention of subjecting ourselves to suffering. Why would someone choose abusive parents knowing they would be abusive? Some believe that we choose the most difficult life experience to elevate ourselves as quickly as possible, but this is not a belief that I subscribe to. In my eyes and from what my spirit guides have conveyed to me, that kind of thing falls under "unknown factors." If you see someone attaining great wealth or it looks like everything is smooth and easy for them, it may simply be their opportunity to "rest" before the next lifetime, in which they'll agree to something more challenging. The way some people talk about "choosing" our lives can verge on victim-blaming, so let me be clear: while our spirit may walk a challenging path with the desire to evolve, we do not choose our suffering.

Reconnecting with my baby from a past life in this one was an opportunity for us to heal and do things differently from before. It gave me a foundation as a parent for understanding where my child may need extra support. It helped me to be prepared for a baby who wouldn't be so keen on strangers or men in general. I wouldn't have a baby who was happy to get passed around the room, as some are. I would have a baby who would need time to warm up and would feel more inclined to be independent when they were reassured that we wouldn't be separated. It was helpful for me to be able to remain grounded in my boundaries around this because I knew it went beyond the usual. Our bond emphasizes why we cannot hold our children choosing us over their heads. We were lucky enough to be chosen; it is a privilege we should treat with honor.

You can learn more through a past-life reading or regression session. In the first, the details of your past life are relayed to you by the reader. In a regression session, you are an active participant. I don't advise doing past-life work via video or prerecorded prompts, because what you experienced might be intense or traumatic. It is critical to have proper guidance so you can have a healing experience, not just get further mired in the trauma. A trained and trustworthy guide can help you understand what your role is or what work needs to be done between you and your baby. They can also help you to better understand your dynamic with each other and how they interact with their siblings.

Here are some things I've learned when it comes to navigating past lives:

Parents and siblings often have a past-life connection, though it isn't always the same relationship they have with each other now. This goes for half siblings and blended families, adopted children, and surrogacy relationships as well. They may have been best friends, one may have been the other's antagonist, or a parent may have been a sibling. The many ways you could have been connected are almost infinite. The thing that these relationships almost always have in common, though, is that in this life they present opportunities for healing—but it's up to you to intuit whether this means fostering togetherness or setting boundaries to protect your family.

You may have heard that a birthmark indicates where you were fatally injured in a past life, but I try not to be so literal about it. Do be mindful of injuries or sensitivities your child may have in that area of the body, which can give insight into a past life—but it is not necessarily a sign of what is to come.

The term "old soul" to refer to a child as someone who has been here before is often weaponized against them. This term tends to be thrown around children who are so "mature" that they take on too many responsibilities before it's age appropriate, which is usually rooted in their inability to depend on others for their needs to be met, or their desire for approval or praise (which they receive when they show they are not "needy"). Independence is one thing, and something all children seek. That isn't the same as not trusting that you can depend on your caretakers to tend to your needs. But there's a truer meaning of this term; old souls are those who have a deep connection to the lives they've lived before, and so have wisdom beyond their years. This wisdom is rooted in meaningful connection (to spirit, nature, and others), kindness, and unconditional love. It's not wisdom related to how to provide for themselves or tend to their own needs because the adults around them don't or can't.

AFFIRMATIONS

- Our past lives are intertwined, but we have a say in how things play out each time.

- I cancel and clear all karmic contracts that cause harm to my baby and me.

- My love for this baby transcends all timelines.

CHAPTER 16

GENDER

We understand there is a spectrum of emotions; why would how we feel about our identity not exist on a spectrum, too?

Your reaction to your baby's biological sex may have been layered—perhaps excitement about certain things to look forward to and concerns, even fears, around the ways the world will treat them based on the box that got checked. (While your child may not grow up to be the sex they were assigned at birth, that doesn't take away from those feelings.) Many parents-to-be, when they're told they are having a girl, become overwhelmed at the thought of the trauma (particularly sexual trauma) that they could experience out in the world. Those who are told they're having a boy, particularly Black and brown parents, may consider how their child will be more likely to experience violence at the hands of police and authority figures, viewed as a man before he has even reached puberty. Others have had a miscarriage and were hoping that the same baby was coming back around, and are disappointed because, to them, this seems to indicate otherwise.

Acceptance is part of healing, and working through our traumas and worries is key to avoiding projecting them onto our children. Healing is a journey that only ends when we have passed on—and even then, we often have work to do. That being said, it's important to address these feelings of gender disappointment privately, with close friends, family, an elder, or a therapist. In the age of social media, when so many of our reactions are preserved for eternity, you never want your child to feel that your love is contingent upon their assigned sex, which could be what they come to believe via the reactions recorded during their gender reveal should they see the footage one day.

I also recommend reflecting on your views and understanding of gender versus sex, sexuality, assigned gender roles, and how to let your child show you who they are and want to be without your projecting or assigning. Journal it out, and consider what it might be like to let a child tell you as they grow. A lot of the time, kids aren't concerned with this until they're older. But you want them to know you are a safe place and refuge when they're trying to figure it out. Journaling can

help you to navigate any feelings that may be in conflict with this by showing you where you may need to
broaden your understanding. For example, if you think
of yourself as pretty open-minded but you aren't comfortable with the idea that Barbie dolls, play makeup,
trucks, and play kitchens are equally appropriate for all
kids, I suggest journaling to reflect on why that is and
what you would be projecting onto your child. They're
simply toys, and an opportunity for children to engage
in play and model behaviors for later in life. It also is
typical of children to want to act out what they see others in their life doing, as a form of play, the same way
they may want an electronic device because they see
how you enjoy being on your phone. Everyone needs to
eat, and cooking is a life skill. We should all be skilled
caretakers, and dolls are an opportunity for practicing
that. Cars and trucks always need fixing, and learning
to drive is a part of life for many people. Playing with
makeup is simply being artistic with a different canvas,
which, considering that almost every kid colors on the
walls at some point, should come as no surprise. You
can continue to expand on these concepts with each
thing that comes up for you. There is magic in getting
our thoughts and feelings out of our heads and onto
paper, where we can reflect on them without feeling
overwhelmed, observe, and come to new conclusions.

When journaling on your personal views regarding gender versus sex, begin by writing out what these terms mean to your personal understanding. Then write out the dictionary definition of each. See how they compare. After, begin to think and write about any ways that, in your own experience, you deviate from those definitions. You may find that, even for you, these terms don't fully encompass how you experience this part of your identity. On a new page, write down what matters most, at the core of your personal values that you hope to convey to your children, such as that they're kind, smart, etc. Notice how these things have no connection to their assigned sex or their gender—or, if you think they do, expand on why you believe that to be so. Continue to do this as you contemplate why you believe this is such an important thing or what impact you believe it will have on them as a whole individual, on their contribution to their community, on their worthiness to be loved by you.

AFFIRMATIONS

- My understanding and beliefs are ever growing.

- My desire to support my child is bigger than my ego.

- I am humbled by the opportunity I have been blessed with to be a parent.

CHAPTER 17

HIGHLY SENSITIVE CHILDREN

W e all are connected. I don't think we should diminish anyone's ability to go beyond the typical human connection of reading someone's facial expressions or sensing when a friend is feeling down, because we know them well. But I also don't believe it makes them special. This is something we all have the ability to tap into; how we do it is what is unique to us.

Many of us understand this concept without realizing it, even if we don't think of ourselves as intuitive people. Consider the phrase "the tension was so thick you could cut it with a knife"; that tension is the energy emitted by our emotions and feelings. We can all turn a radio dial and tune in to different stations, and while most are vibing out to FM, we can all switch to AM with a press of a button. Some of us are more practiced at listening to both on a daily basis, but it is something all of us can do.

Babies and toddlers read our energy as a means of survival and bonding. They recognize who is safe based on energy, tone, and other nonverbal cues. How this shows up varies for everyone. As a toddler, I was referred to as a "selective talker." I would chat up my parents, but I would not talk to most people. While some credited this to being shy, it wasn't that. My parents were a source of calm, grounding, safe energy for me, whereas much of the rest of the world often felt overwhelming. My dad never yelled and always said, "I won't raise my voice with you until you're old and hard of hearing." My mom could be stern if needed, but she never yelled, either (until I was older and doing wild shit I wasn't supposed to). Being quiet was my way of grounding myself, at an age when I was too young to have the tools I would later learn. I modeled what my parents did, in the way a toddler could. Being quiet also allowed me to take in what was happening around me, who was safe, who wasn't. The other side to this is that I didn't exchange energy with just anybody. We all respond differently and engage differently, because of what's modeled for us, our experiences, and our personality.

Something then happens to most—but not all—of us as we get older: we stop listening to both sides of the radio. Between the way society operates in favor of disconnection and the narrative many of us hear that rejects this way of being, it is no surprise that many stop listening to both. That is, unless we remain highly sensitive. If you have a highly sensitive kid, you probably know it. They often look like a child who sees shadows where others don't (outside of any actual physiological vision issues); can sense when something is wrong; tells you about the spirits—and is clear that they are not "imaginary friends"; explains past lives they've experienced; and may be labeled "difficult" or "moody." They "feel too much."

All children have their challenges, they just differ from child to child. Which is why the question is how you can best support your child and honor their talents, even if you don't fully understand them.

"Highly sensitive" is a term that can be used in regard to both emotion and energy. For some, the activation of this ability is rooted in trauma and learning to survive. It can look like hyper-focusing on the emotions and needs of others to the point where you make them your responsibility, or catering to someone to avoid abuse or to establish yourself as "important" to them. For others, it is an ability that they didn't leave behind in childhood for other reasons.

Being supportive of highly sensitive children can

feel overwhelming, from the reminder of the trauma we experienced in childhood at the hands of others to the overstimulation that can occur for parents. It's critical to be gentle with ourselves and them. To extend grace to both. Children are learning how to exist in this realm (even if they've been here before, they're still starting from scratch in many ways), and we are learning how to be parents. Modeling many times over how to regulate their emotions and simply observe others' energy, rather than taking it on, is an ongoing act. You do this by regulating your own emotions and modeling ways to observe, not absorb.

Start by creating routines that aren't limited to the bedtime wind-down but are centered in cleansing energy or emotionally checking in. That can look like giving them herbal or spiritual baths, such as the ones mentioned in chapter 9, on a weekly basis; giving them a kid-safe energetic spray to use if they feel uncomfortable while they're out of the house; dusting them with cascarilla before they go out for the day; or teaching them grounding meditations. Even simple techniques, such as 5-4-3-2-1 (see page 161), can bring you back to the present and tune you back in to your own body. This can be a way to help them identify when they are tuning in to the feelings of others as opposed to their own.

Try making a kid-safe energetic spray with equal parts rosemary, basil, sage, bay leaf, and frankincense hydrosol. Have them mist themselves with it and make sweeping motions downward to cleanse. They can do this before leaving the house, before coming inside the home, and anytime while they're out. If you'd prefer a simpler option, give them a spray bottle of rosewater that they can do the same with. As they grow older, have them use simple affirmations while they do this, such as "I am cleansed of all negative energies" or "I am cleansed of all energies that are not mine." Help them to create affirmations of their own that they feel good about saying. Be proactive with them. Have them use an emotions chart to identify their feelings, and ask if this is how they themselves feel or how they feel because of what others around them are feeling. This can be another way to teach them about taking on the emotions of others as their own early on.

Bring them into your own energetic hygiene routine. By doing this, you're modeling healthy self-care and setting up a foundation that will support them and their sensitivities.

If your child is very sensitive emotionally but their reactiveness is not activated by others' energy, consider helping them create rituals around navigating their feelings—such as learning to pause, productively expressing their emotions, and finding their voice—by modeling those behaviors. Children learn how to speak up for themselves when they see their parents doing it; same with learning how to pause and express their emotions. Affirm and guide them to do it in a way that feels comfortable for them. Help your child understand that the uncomfortable emotions are just as important to feel as the comfortable ones. Learning to sit with them is what helps us get to the other side. What we do with those feelings is what makes a difference.

When you feel your own emotions rearing up, as they do for all of us, remind yourself:

- We're learning together in the school of life.

- My child is a tiny person with big emotions, which can be overwhelming for them.

- My child feels safest with me, which can sometimes lead to them be explosive—because they know I will not leave them. I can help them regulate. I am their safe space.

Keeping your home as close to a sanctuary as possible is important not just for your sensitive child but for you, too. Tending to its energy is part of that. Do your best to keep clutter to a minimum so energy flows freely and doesn't become stagnant, cleanse your space regularly, and have plants that raise the vibration and air quality. Unwelcome energy will inevitably come into your home at times, but you can make an effort to prevent it. Hanging bells on your door or doorknob clears energy before it enters your home and is thought to keep low-vibrational spirits away; keeping a rosemary or rue plant in a pot at your front door offers protection as well. So does keeping aloe, a snake plant, and other plants in the home. Teach your children to be kind to them, and support them in building a relationship with them. Plants will take a hit for you if someone sends something your way, especially when you have a solid relationship. This is also why it's important to teach children to respect, be kind to, and be loving of things that aren't human. They're our siblings, from the same Mother Nature.

While not everyone works with archangels and saints, we all can call on protective spirits in times of need. Teach your child to call on protective forces, whether it's Archangel Michael/Saint Michael, their ancestors, their spirit guides, another saint or deity, or a higher power. This is particularly beneficial for highly sensitive children, because so much of what they experience is not something everyone around them will understand. Knowing that they have allies even in the unseen helps them understand they are never alone.

If working with something that is faith or energy based doesn't resonate, I encourage you to consider a psychological approach. But don't ignore or try to pretend this experience isn't happening; these things don't just go away, and your little one deserves support navigating what they're experiencing.

Indigo Water

Keeping a regularly changed bowl of indigo water around can shift the energy of your home, bringing in peace and tranquility. Use indigo water to cleanse a space, by either dousing your front entrance or adding it to your floor wash to mop with. While this formula can vary from practitioner to practitioner, the basics are below.

Clear glass bowl

Enough cool water to fill the bowl to the brim

1 squirt of liquid bluing or 1 laundry bluing block/ball

1 camphor/alcanfor tablet

Sprinkle of cascarilla

Optional: alum/alumbre; Florida water or holy water

Note: Keep out of reach of children; this is toxic if consumed. Pregnant people should avoid camphor or burning camphor tablets/oil because inhaling large amounts isn't safe. There is debate about whether it's safe to use topically, so you can wear sterile gloves to handle the tablet, then remove them. The camphor is very diluted in the water, and the vapors aren't directly inhaled because you are not using hot water.

Combine cool water and the bluing in a bowl. You can also grate the bluing for easier absorption; just use a grater that's not used for food. Add the camphor tablet and mix until well combined. Sprinkle in the cascarilla. Stir. If you want to add alum, simply place a chunk in the bowl. You can add a splash of Florida water or holy water if you feel called to, but not everyone does. Pray over it and speak in your intentions. Pray for peace, calm, and tranquility to fill the home, and for protection from negative energy, energetic attacks, and the evil eye/mal de ojo. Place the bowl either by the entrance of your home (preferred) or in the center of your home.

....

HERBAL SUGGESTIONS

- **Rosewater:** Use as a spray or add to baths for protection.

- **Chamomile:** Make an infusion and add to baths for cleansing.

- **Lavender:** Add to bathwater or use in body products for protection. Dried lavender can also be placed in a sachet under your child's pillow or hung above your baby's crib or bed for protection and to keep away nightmares.

- **Calendula:** Make an infusion and add to baths for strength. Put blossoms in a sachet to ward off nightmares or to give strength and protection.

- **Basil:** Add to baths or energetic sprays.

- **Rosemary:** Add to baths or energetic sprays, or burn to cleanse their space.

- **Violet:** Add violet cologne to baths for tranquility and emotional balance.

- **Cascarilla:** Add to baths. Use to make a protective marking, such as a simple + or X, on children for protection, or dust them with it.

- **Camphor:** Place a tablet in a glass bowl of water along with alum to protect and cleanse a bedroom.

- **Elderflower:** Place in sachets and hang above doorways to offer protection. Add to baths to break hexes.

AFFIRMATIONS

- My child's sensitivity is a gift that I honor.

- My child's ability to read others is to be respected.

- I welcome the opportunity to be my child's ally.

CHAPTER 18

A WORD FROM TWO WISE MOTHERS

Parenthood can feel lonely, and not everyone has the same access when it comes to connecting with others who can give them guidance or support. Finding elders whose vibe resonates with our heart isn't always easy, either. But they're worth seeking out. Wisdom and support from those who have walked before us can be such a helpful part of our experience. None of us are born knowing everything, and we won't learn it all in one lifetime. With shared wisdom, we are more likely to make better-informed choices. You'll still make mistakes, but it can help you to feel confident in your ability to handle the aftermath. Knowing this, I wanted to share insight from two seasoned moms who are spiritual practitioners as well. They are also two elders in my life who have both helped me navigate this human experience as a spiritual being, motherhood, and more. Sometimes people no longer have their mothers, grandmothers, or mother figures, or never did. Stepping into parenthood can feel so lonely and scary without them. While these wise words cannot replace that relationship, I hope they give some comfort and solid guidance for those who need it.

Yvonne Secreto has been a blessing in my life and in the lives of many others. She is a registered nurse and a practitioner of past-life regression, inner-child work, Reiki, and more. She has supported my own personal growth, healing, and spiritual development. Below is one of her experiences as a mother and spiritual practitioner, coupled with advice on navigating these kinds of situations with your children.

"Mommy, Mommy, there's something in my room!"

I chuckled as my nine-year-old daughter came running down the stairs. "I'm sorry, it's your great-great-grandmother." She had visited me (as she always does) while I was cleaning up the kitchen, and I'd asked her to wait for me upstairs.

"WHAT! Are you crazy? You sent a spirit to my room!"

"First of all, our grammy brings us gifts when she visits, and she loves and protects us."

I knew at that moment that it was time to start teaching her about spiritual protection.

"There are rules in the unseen just like there are rules in our visible day-to-day lives. Any time you sense a spirit, you have the right to determine if it stays in your space or not. Always make the statement 'You must leave if you are not of the light.' Invoking the light will immediately raise the vibratory frequency around you so that anything that is negative cannot tolerate the energy, and it will naturally dissipate or leave. When you call the light into the room or around your body, you are always protected."

She listened intently, and throughout the years, she has given me many, many examples of positive outcomes despite brushes with danger because she invoked the light.

—Yvonne Secreto

Iya Michelle Hunton was brought into my life not too long after I had my firstborn. She is a formidable force for kindness, love, strength, and wisdom. I have called on her many times when I was in need, and I knew when writing this book that others would benefit greatly from what she has to share. While I may not be an authority figure in regard to what she shares, she most certainly is. Below she has shared some of her personal experience as a mother and guidance that we can all take away.

When each person is born on this earth, we come equipped with our personal inner knowing. This is the part of a person that is connected to God or is God. How you conduct your life does not matter. Your inner knowing will never leave you. Many people refer to it as their first mind. This God connection lives in our head and in our gut. As a mother, this voice tends to get louder. Some people may call it instinct. It is your inner knowing.

When I had my first son, my mother gave me some sound advice. She said to listen to the doctor. That's good, but never dismiss what your head and your gut are telling you about your baby. My mother called it "mother wit"; she said nothing beats mother wit.

Children don't come with a guide to tell us how to rear, protect, and teach them. But mothers do have mother wit, or our inner knowing, speaking to us.

I was a single mother with two sons three years apart, divorcing my husband. I was unhappy. But one thing was clear to me. I had to make sound choices for my children. My needs were secondary. I understood that if I put the work in on these children, if I did everything that I could to give them a good life, they could become great citizens in this world. I also knew that if I neglected to do this, they would become a liability to this world. So I made the choice to give it the best I had for as long as I could. I was blessed, because they turned out to be great citizens.

I wish I could say I had knowledge of how to bring them up, but I didn't. I did know that voice. That voice that would speak to me and let me know when they were in danger or about to face a problem. I didn't have a lot of resources, but I did know how to pray. I taught my sons how to pray.

Each and every day, before we left our house, we would join hands and say a prayer. We prayed that we'd return home without hurt, harm, or danger. God honored that prayer, and we are grateful.

My circumstances were not normal. When I left that marriage, my ex-husband was so angry that I would leave and take my children. The abuse became worse, even deadly. They told me he would shoot me in open court. Therefore, praying to come home each day was serious business for my little family. I did not want my sons to fear, but I wanted them to live well, to be happy, to enjoy their childhood. So I had to become very spiritual. I had to listen to that voice, and if my head and guts said, "No, don't go," we didn't go.

If my head said, "Get in the car and ride until you are safe," that's what we did. I think the greatest gift out of this horrible circumstance was my teaching my sons about faith, God, and perseverance.

Any time I felt my children were being affected by the drama, I would clean them with something. It could be candy, fruit, bread. I took the item and rubbed the top of their heads, back of their necks, chest areas (especially the heart areas), arms, and legs, then threw it in the trash. This helped them not to internalize any negativity.

—Iya Michelle Hunton

As I've said before, take what you need and leave what you don't. But know that these are words from the heart.

AFFIRMATIONS

- I possess the ability to connect with the elders I need to be my guides through motherhood.

- I am open to receiving the wisdom of those who have honored this calling before me.

- I am blessed to sit at the feet of elders who support me and my baby.

AFTERWORD

This book began when I was pregnant with my first-born and has been a labor of love in the making since then. I will admit that it has been one of the hardest things I have done in this lifetime. I don't believe myself to be an authority figure in this life—though younger me may have at one time. I'm simply a mom sharing things that have helped me and others. I pray that in these chapters, you, too, have found something that helps you or someone you love through the wild ride. Too often in today's society, birthing parents are made to feel forgotten, discarded, or pushed out, which breaks the tradition of supporting them through their initiation into parenthood. Let this be a reminder to bring back the tradition of communal love and support. A push to support those in your life who become pregnant after you or at the same time, even if you're miles apart. Share the knowledge you've gained, the way the women in chapter 18 have. Set the tone. We are the future ancestors, and so are our little ones.

ACKNOWLEDGMENTS

Thank you to my parents and my ancestors who came before them. Without you, I wouldn't even exist. Thank you to the father of my children, CJ, for choosing to embark on this wild journey called parenthood with me. As you say, "We dropped the dopest mixtape." For me, we created magic in a world that can sometimes feel empty of that. Thank you to my elders for blessing me with the privilege of having them in my life. Thank you to my guides; without them, I wouldn't have the words to fill these pages.

RESOURCES

Blogs and Websites

originalbotanica.com

cafeastrology.com

Sancista Brujo Luis YouTube Channel: https://www
.youtube.com/channel/UCakUvflW5-Vk9iXPkWStyGw

Books

Cunningham's Encyclopedia of Magical Herbs by Scott
Cunningham

*Earth and Spirit: Medicinal Plants and Healing Lore from
Puerto Rico* by Maria Benedetti